The
Stress Elimination
Handbook

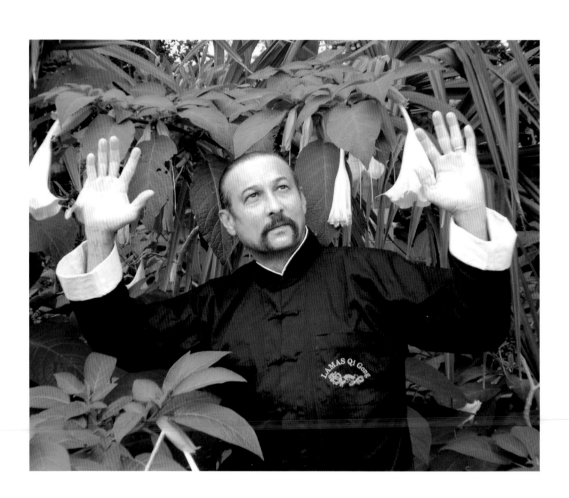

THE
STRESS ELIMINATION
HANDBOOK

A holistic self-help program to restore health,
achieve balance, and promote well-being

GRANDMASTER
ADRIAN SIMON LOWE

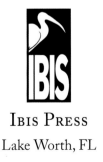

IBIS PRESS
Lake Worth, FL

Published in 2010 by Ibis Press
An imprint of Nicolas-Hays, Inc.
P.O. Box 540206
Lake Worth, FL 33454-0206
www.nicolashays.com

Distributed to the trade by
Red Wheel/Weiser, LLC
65 Parker St., Ste. 7
Newburyport, MA 01950
www.redwheelweiser.com

ISBN 978-089254-162-1

Library of Congress Cataloging-in-Publication Data

Lowe, Adrian Simon.
  The stress elimination handbook : a holistic self-help program to restore
health,   achieve balance, and promote well-being / Adrian Simon Lowe.
     p. cm.
  ISBN 978-0-89254-162-1 (alk. paper)
  1. Stress management. 2. Qi gong. 3. Relaxation. I. Title.
  RA785.L69 2010
  613.7'9—dc22   2010021735

Book design and production by Studio 31
www.studio31.com

Photos of Grandmaster Lowe demonstrating
the Lion Tail Qi Gong positions by Julia Pineda

Photo of Jefferson Memorial (page 137) by Rachel Wasserman

16 15 14 13 12 11 10
 7   6   5   4   3   2   1

Printed in China

Acknowledgements

I WISH TO THANK my dear wife Diane for her patience and the months she spent proofreading. Most importantly, for the many long years she has stood by, waiting uncomplainingly while I was teaching, guiding and helping others—thereby sorely neglecting our own family with my sporadic and protracted absences.

Secondly, to all those good and forward-thinking people, who have become more aware of how to care for their personal health and who, by their individual joyful experiences, have increased their determination to progress in their journey toward ever improving good health.

My objective in writing this material was to ensure that all people have the opportunity to enhance and maintain their personal health if they so desire and thereby lead a more Spiritually rewarding life.

My passion is to make as many individuals as possible aware of the powerful Chinese Healing Art of Qi Gong. Thus, wherever possible, to provide a simple means by which they can obtain information and learn of my traditional family art, namely LAMAS Qi Gong, The Ancient Chinese Healing Art.

This book is my humble attempt to offer readers an easy and simple means to gaining insights, skills and knowledge to make life easier and more rewarding.

Table of Contents

Part Four: More on Qi Gong

Appendices

A Word on Stress

Stress is a fact of modern life. Depending on the type of activity in which you may be involved, some aspects of that endeavor are likely to trigger the onset of stress.

Stress knows few boundaries and occurs during many sorts of physical work, sports and even during moments of enjoyment. Stress may also occur while performing daily chores and of course, during cerebral activities.

One may experience stress while involved in research, attending a conference, providing entertainment, or merely socializing. Whether you are young or old, stress respects no one.

The onset of stress-related illness is invasive and insidious. Its effects may take many years to reveal themselves, or may attack a person within minutes, establishing almost instantaneous symptomology.

My purpose in writing this book is to provide tried and tested self-help measures for any forward-thinking individual. This book is designed to offer easy-to-follow instructions to control, manage, reduce and eliminate stress.

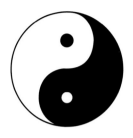

Part One:

Understanding Stress

Tribal Lore Leads the Way to Health

Lore from my ancestors had been handed down only through an oral tradition among tribal family members. One such story recounts how some members of the LoLo, one of the most ancient tribes of China, were outdoors one particularly dreary, chilly afternoon thousands of years ago.

The family huddled around a fire that provided warmth and light, and allowed them to cook their food. They noticed that the steam rising from the food in the pot, when blown by a gentle breeze in one particular direction, seemed to cast a wave-like image.

Knowing that food was vital for life, my ancestors drew three wavy lines depicting the image they saw.

These three slanting wavy lines represent the life force or Qi (pronounced *chi*) of the food. Each line symbolizes one of the Three Treasures: *Shen, Qi* and *Jing*, or Spirit, Mind and Body.

These wavy lines became the first Chinese character to depict this power, this Qi.

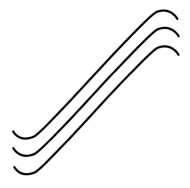

Qi is in all of nature and can be cultivated with the daily practice of LAMAS Qi Gong. (Subsequently, to be referred to as Qi Gong.)

Could my ancestors have predicted that their understanding of Qi would eventually be passed along to individuals like you in the 21st century—people yearning for well-being, improved health and a well-balanced life?

Hopefully, one would like to think that they did.

* * *

Stress has its roots in the very essence of life and has caused more suffering and diminishment of the human spirit than any other form of affliction.

As an Empath and holistic healer, I've witnessed the effects of stress on innumerable individuals, their families, broader society and generally, most communities in our world.

Without a doubt, I know that stress is the surest way to become a victim of future ill health. Hence, I am revealing what was once esoteric knowledge, and core wisdom that was not previously available.

This book will provide you with more than a mere understanding of stress. It is my personal, detailed analysis of stress and its harmful and even deadly effects on the strength of the human spirit, the conscious and subconscious levels of mental endurance and on the efficacy of our bodily systems.

The information and techniques presented here are steps along the path to a longer and improved quality of life.

I encourage you to follow this path. It is the Way by which you may prolong and enjoy your life and its rich, meaningful, rewarding and dynamic experiences.

Qi Gong is your path to reduce, prevent and eliminate stress. Practice will heighten your awareness. Moreover, it is possible to find real peace and true harmony within yourself.

A constant in our daily lives, stress weakens Qi and is the genesis of disease. Change is also a constant in our daily existence.

Therefore, to change the impact and damage caused by stress, we need to purposefully and diligently employ another constant factor to prevent stress.

What is this constant factoring that which we must use? It is Qi, our life force.

This book provides you with accurate and easy-to-follow instructions that will allow and help you to regenerate your Qi and re-orient your life force.

By reading and following the methods which I outline here, you will be taking the first very real steps in accepting responsibility for the direction of your health in the near and distant future.

This is a profound decision on your part and the results can also have a dramatic impact, because stress has ubiquitous effects that can swamp your internal biotic defenses.

Our aim should be to allow our lives to reflect divine harmony. This is the true goal of the cultivation of Qi, as will be explained.

But first, we must understand our enemy: Stress.

The Enemy Attacks Before Birth

"I AM SO STRESSED OUT," is a typical phrase uttered by millions of people both yesterday and today and will be repeated by millions more tomorrow. This common statement is usually made in an attempt to describe a state of being low in energetic potential.

Surprisingly, we first experienced stress long before we ever struggled with school, work or complex relationships. In fact, we actually endured stress even before we were born.

The effects of stress have become so prevalent in modern society that even the mainstream press has been forced to recognize the problem. Throughout this book, I will refer to articles in popular publications to help emphasize the ubiquitous nature of this phenomena.

For example, in an article entitled "Mother's Stress Puts Baby at Risk of Schizophrenia," published in the *Daily Mail* (U.K., February 5, 2008), medical correspondent Jenny Hope described a study published in the Archives of Psychiatry at the Manchester research center of Tommy's (the baby charity that funded the study). Researchers concluded that babies whose mothers suffered severe stress in the first three months of pregnancy, "may be at risk of schizophrenia."

They defined severe stress to include such issues as the death or severe illness of a close relative or loved one. The study concluded that children whose mothers had experienced such traumas, were sixty-seven percent more like to suffer from schizophrenia in later life.

Schizophrenia is a mental health disorder whose symptoms include hallucinations, delusions, and rapid mood changes. The article quoted Professor Philip Baker, of Tommy's, "Increasingly we are learning that the environment a baby is exposed to inside the womb is determining its long-term health."

Thus, the early months of pregnancy, often ignored and considered of little consequence, are indeed an important determinant of a successful pregnancy. Jenny Hope further quoted Professor Baker's statement, "These are quite new concepts but they are really changing the way we think about pregnancy and much more longer-term effects on a baby's health."

While the article cautioned that expectant mothers should not become over-anxious about their pregnancies, it is my belief that our basic existence is affected even at conception. I contend that there is a conditioning struggle for life itself.

After conception, the fetus is subjected to the same levels and types of stress as the mother, due to daily occurrences and events and her efforts to face life's demands and challenges. Therefore, if the mother-to-be is experiencing a difficult time during pregnancy, regardless of the cause, the unborn infant will innately and instinctively sense most of the various bio-chemical changes and psychodynamics, (interaction of emotional forces) and the myriad emotional disturbances and challenges engineered by stress.

Because of this perspicacity (acute perception), the unborn infant will be prenatally programmed with the stress-generating hormone and hence, its habituation. This creates a cause and effect relationship that medical studies have further corroborated.

This aspect is discussed in another article in the *Daily Mail*, on March 31, 2008. Science reporter Fiona MacRae reported on a study conducted by the Edinburgh University regarding the issue of pre-natal stress. Here, excessive stress suffered by the mother during pregnancy was documented to create the risk of heart disease and diabetes later in life.

The stress hormone cortisol was considered responsible. Scientists believe that high cortisol production may be responsible for altering the proper function of the genes. Thus, they postulated that grandchildren may be at risk as well.

This study expanded the range of stress factors to include pressures at work, financial fears, marital difficulties and "anxiety about pregnancy itself."

Fiona MacRae reported that previous research had also linked maternal stress to later childhood problems of hyperactivity and other emotional problems.

I believe that the perturbations occurring within our human system, cause the initial chemical onset of stress. The characteristic by which hormone production may be viewed, is as a chemical substance in the body's endocrine glands, or certain other cells that exert a regulatory or stimulatory effect. A typical example is in the process of metabolism.

Another recent article, published in the April 6, 2010 edition of the *Daily Mail,* written by David Derbyshire, is headlined, "Drinking in pregnancy 'puts baby at risk of epilepsy.'" Researchers found that children exposed to alcohol while in the womb were more likely to suffer from seizures as they matured. Derbyshire quantifies the problem with these statistics. Four hundred twenty-five people were studied who suffer from FASD (Fetal Alcohol Spectrum Disorder). The subjects were between the ages of two and forty-nine. While only one percent of all people develop epilepsy, six percent of those with FASD had been diagnosed with epilepsy. Of those, twelve percent had experienced at least one seizure.

The article quotes Dr. Dan Savage, a neuroscientist at the University of New Mexico. "This report builds on a growing body of evidence that maternal drinking during pregnancy may put a child at greater risk for an even wider variety of neurological and behavioral health problems than we appreciated before. The consensus recommendation of scientists and clinical investigators, along with public health officials around the world, is very clear—a woman should abstain from drinking during pregnancy as part of an overall program of good prenatal care."

Derbyshire mentions that past studies have shown FASD causes attention deficit disorder, hyperactivity, and poor manual coordination. It also puts people at greater risk of later developing alcoholism, drug abuse, and depression. Finally, the British National Institute of Health and Clinical Excellence cautioned the public about the risk of miscarriage caused by alcohol related stress during the first three months of pregnancy.

If we are under stress prior to our actual birth during development in the womb, then it is self-evident that we will be born with the problems associated with stress. Furthermore, if we can regard the internal environment as stress-causing, it is reasonable to assume that the external environment will also cause stress.

We can categorize stress as either internal or external.

External causes of stress include poverty, extreme temperature variations, physical trauma, microbes (germs), all types of pollution, prenatal and postnatal conditions and fear.

Other types of internal causes of stress are genetic weakness, sexual excess, overeating, lack of exercise and again, fear.

Anger is one significant stress condition. This state of stress has a rather disturbing effect on the liver since anger is of an emotional content and as such, has a connection to liver disharmony. Whereas at other times, stress may make one feel helpless or ill at ease and can even bring on periods of extreme fatigue.

Stress is a constant factor throughout our lifetime. The lifecycle transitions between childhood, adolescence and into adulthood constantly place us in stressful situations. This is true at our work and even in our play. Whatever the type of pastime or hobby we enjoy, be it group exercise or individual sport, whether combative, sedentary or vigorous, elements of stress are constantly introduced. Whether we enjoy what we are doing or not, we must accept that most of our actions generate some level of stress. Yes, those include even our pleasures!

Improper food including sugar and artificial sweeteners, fast foods, packaged, tinned, canned or boxed foods, excessive acidic or acid-producing foods, caffeine and alcohol are all contributors to stress, as are smoking and secondary smoke. Add to these, excessive work pressures caused by long hours without necessary breaks and competitive struggles to be at the same level as others. Additional factors including: domestic issues, peer pressures, pregnancy, environmental toxins, media, competition, lack of exercise, prescription and non-prescription drugs, excessive reading, talking, gambling and violence of any description provide a recipe for damage to the spirit, mind and body. All of these eventually lead to illness, disease and in many instances, even to preventable death!

As though stress is vindictive, the ailments it spawns will eventually strike us in a way that we cannot ignore, hitting us where it matters most and often, when we expect it least. The stealth effects of stress were illustrated in an interesting story in the *Daily Mail* (February 12, 2008). Adrian Monti, the Good Health columnist, wrote, "Last April, L. C. stood before thousands of pop fans at Wembley arena in London as they waited for her to sing. But as she opened her mouth she discovered that she had lost her voice. The singer, whose distinctive voice has won plaudits from Mika and Rod Stewart, was supporting the chart-topping Sugababes on tour."

The article explained that the singer was suffering from severe acid reflux which had "burnt" her vocal cords. It explained that certain foods—especially acidic or spicy meals, chocolate or particularly fatty or rich foods, can cause the diaphragmatic sphincter to relax, allowing stomach acids to rise up the esophagus, especially when a person is lying down. The diaphragmatic sphincter is also affected by smoking, alcohol and stress. As a result of the acid, the esophagus becomes inflamed and swollen.

Typical symptoms include heartburn, which is pain in the upper chest or abdomen, as well as nausea, a need to belch, accompanied by an acidic taste in the mouth, or "huskiness" in the voice. The article explained that L.C. had probably unknowingly suffered acid reflux for years but may not have had any other obvious symptoms. It was the intense use of her voice during performances that exacerbated the problem.

Adrian Monti also claimed that acid reflux is on the rise and that many doctors believe it to be caused by our changing modern lifestyle. The reporter quotes Dr. Simon Gabe, senior gastroenterologist at St. Marks Hospital in Harrow, North-West London. "It's a disease, which is clearly on the rise in the Western world. And it seems to be the usual causes—obesity, too much alcohol and a lack of exercise—which are to blame. The patients I see are only the tip of the iceberg."

Monti continues that while changes in lifestyle are an effective means of helping most people, too many patients seek a medicinal solution instead. The article explains that alternatives to medicine include simple solutions like reducing fatty food intake and thinking carefully about meal times. For example, eating late at night and then going to bed causes food to lodge within the digestive tract and remain improperly digested. "Aim to eat three to four hours before going to bed, cut down on alcohol and smoking, also take more regular exercise."

You'll note the irony that many of the substances in which people indulge to reduce stress actually worsen it, robbing the spirit, mind and body of the opportunity to heal itself.

Some typical stress-related complaints will also be found in a culture that may be lacking in spiritually. As we have seen, the sources of stress are endless.

Stress manifests itself in varied ways and in clinically dissimilar stages, producing apparently non-connected signs or symptoms.

Some symptoms suffered due to stressful experiences may include:

- Irritable Bowel Syndrome
- Chronic skin conditions
- Bloating
- Abdominal pains
- Loss of short-term memory
- Feeling emotionally and physically overwhelmed
- Chronic anxiety and panic attacks

- Extreme fatigue
- Lack of coherence in daily life
- Psycho-social complaints
- Inability to cope with mundane and complex tasks
- Scoliosis can be aggravated
- Immune system diseases
- Organ failure

The daily pressures that cause stress can quickly drain our reserves of strength and energy. Furthermore, there is fallout to others. Those who maintain contact with individuals under stress will eventually suffer similar conditions themselves. These may include friends, family, co-workers and even such casual levels of contact as waitresses, police and others.

There will also be occasions of frustration, apart from the dysfunctional factors associated with being in a stressed condition. Stress can delay the improvement of health and in most cases, causes deterioration, in spite of the best conventional medical treatments available.

One perceives the various stages of stress, then tries to react accordingly in an effort to cope with these internal dysfunctional pressures. However, it is apparent that the human system cannot independently alleviate or eliminate the damaging and insidious condition commonly known as stress.

A person will experience the effects of stress even before one notices an ailment dire enough to be called an illness or disease by conventional terms. It is likely that anyone under stress will suffer from the loss of physical well-being and will experience a reduced mental capacity. Often the term "stress" is employed to depict those who seem to have a depressed or disenchanted human Spirit.

Stress is and will always be the most damaging life factor:

- Stress produces a feeling of isolation.
- Stress produces a sense of loss of direction.
- Stress induces a fear factor, which in itself can be alarming.
- Whether you are young or old, stress affects everyone, regardless of your age.
- Stress affects us all, regardless of our gender, religious beliefs and state of health.
- No amount of wealth or public esteem can dissuade an attack of stress.
- Stress is the one factor that will eventually affect your health, financial status, the way you think and behave, and therefore your overall quality of life, including your longevity.
- In fact, stress has already affected you even if you have no signs or symptoms.
- Stress deprives us of the very essence of good health.
- Stress reduces and destroys our Qi levels.
- Stress restricts our Qi flow.
- Restricted Qi flow causes unsmooth Qi flow.
- Unsmooth Qi Flow causes organ deficiency.
- Organs that are deficient or have restricted Qi flow will become diseased.

We cannot leave it to chance to learn how the Spirit-Mind-Body connection must handle stress. This is why I have written this book. Learn how to combat stress, and you can reach the top of your game.

What is Stress?

My personal description of stress is as follows:

> Stress is pressure or tension exerted on a substance, material, or object making demands of a physical nature. The mechanical force of stress manifests as force per unit area between contiguous bodies or parts of a body. Stress exerts pressure or tension through eight different avenues of our spiritual, mental and physical selves.

These eight avenues when impacted by stress or stimuli are affected as follows:

1. Emotional conditions
2. Physical, mental, or physiological conditions
3. Debilitation or exhaustion
4. Chemical reactions
5. Psychologically dysfunctional behaviors
6. Mental and physical tension
7. The onset of illness or disease
8. Thermal reactions

The stress response in the human body can involve more than 1,400 physical and chemical reactions. By these numbers alone, you can imagine the problems which may arise because of so many different chemical changes occurring in the blink of an eye. Add to that, the fact that the stress response also activates more than thirty different neurotransmitters that release various harmful hormones. Clearly, it is evident that the excessive release of "stress hormones" will damage cells, tissues and organs. Therefore, it is reasonable to conclude that stress is the original cause of disease.

Stress damages the human body. It disrupts the flow of our life essence, or Qi, and will eventually compromise our health.

Think of your typical day and all the stress you are subjected to. We will be exposed to some form of stress when we communicate with family members, friends or even complete strangers. Moreover, there will be rudimentary and supplementary pressures that are sure to be part of that experience.

Imagine that stress is opening a spigot, releasing an incessant drip of disease-causing stress hormones. The reactions to those hormones occur not only in the body tissue, but also in the system's functioning and the brain itself.

Attempting to internalize stress, by keeping signs or symptoms within oneself, or ignoring stress by behaving and or pretending that there is really nothing wrong, can cause even greater damage than an occasional, though traumatic experience.

Please read the previous sentence again.

The elimination of such stressors as alcohol, smoking, fast foods and the external causes of stress previously listed, will provide benefits and some noticeable changes. But there is more to the stress story than merely giving up bad habits.

Negative thoughts too, are bio-chemically produced energies that will become destructive.

Since emotions and stress are interwoven, one should strive to think good thoughts, say good words, perform acts of kindness and do well.

Best of all, stress is avoidable through the practice of Lion's Tail Qi Gong (LAMAS ShiQi).

Fight or Flight: The Adrenaline Cascade

THERE ARE FIVE EMOTIONAL PATTERNS that provoke the onset of stress.

We are rarely consciously able to make use of, or are even aware of these five responses. In fact, at every level they are all emotionally driven and have different effects on us during the course of our entire lifespan.

They are woven into the fabric of our very existence. Each of the five emotional patterns is associated with an invasive and destructive nature. All are stress orientated.

As you read about the emotional patterns and the organ connections that can become damaged, think of your emotions. What is your dominant emotional state? Later in this book, you will learn how to prevent further damage caused by emotive patterns.

Traditional Chinese Medicine views the body, the organs and their interrelationships, systems and symptoms differently from Western medicine, as you'll note in the paired organs below.

1. ANGER damages the Liver-Heart connection, producing a breath said to be uneven and rough.
2. ENVY causes a breath that injures the Heart-Spleen connection and has an emotional discord.
3. WORRY attacks the Spleen-Lungs connection, causing depression, while inducing shallow non-beneficial breathing.
4. FEAR, the most damaging emotional state, destroys the Lungs-Kidney connection and negates nourishment of all the other Yin/Yang Organs (more on that later). Fear is the great inhibitor and disrupter of smooth Qi flow.

5. CONFLICT, the usurper of the Kidney-Liver connection, is instrumental in causing humans to become the worst type of primitive savages, while pretending that the conflict is for the common good. Conflict results in a short, sharp pattern of breathing.

Each of the emotive patterns results in a deviant breathing pattern, which in turn, initiates a release of adrenaline.

A slow drip of adrenaline will inevitably set off symptoms of anxiety to be visibly displayed and noticeable to others. However, the sufferer would experience some forms of discomfort even before obvious signals have become noticeable. The degree of this state of un-ease, will depend on the type and severity of the problem that initially triggered the signs of anxiety.

When we are faced with stressful moments, our fight or flight reflexes, which are our main survival mechanisms, will cause and create a release of the hormones adrenalin and cortisol. These increase the pulse rate of the heart, which in turn gives the body and brain an energetic boost. Muscles will tense and cholesterol is released into the blood stream.

This chain reaction is a protective measure to make our blood clot more easily in case of injuries or wounds. Under normal conditions, the flight or flight response gives us the extra energy needed to save both our lives and those of others in specific dangerous situations, such as escaping a burning building or combating an enemy.

On the contrary, in today's stressful environment, we generally don't expend the energy boost necessary for fleeing a burning building or fighting the enemy. Although we are stressed, it is usually not because a hostile individual, nor what are commonly termed "bad people," are attacking us.

The chain reaction of survival mechanisms can trigger health complaints, including but not limited to:

- Heart attacks
- Strokes
- Cancers
- Stomach ulcers
- Alzheimer's disease
- Schizophrenia

An adrenaline rush will trigger a panic attack. Subsequently, this panic attack produces a fear factor in the person concerned. Hence, it is logical to follow this chain of events: the increased flow of adrenaline produces fear and consequently makes the individual feel even more stressed.

I term this increased flow, "adrenaline cascade." (See flow chart).

In addition, uncertainty—be it on a mental level, caused by a physical dysfunction, or even a lack of spirituality, can significantly increase the flow of adrenaline, thus resulting in stress.

How are we able overcome this particular form of stress caused by an excess of adrenaline?

Examining the fact that shallow breathing or taking short breaths produces an increased adrenaline flow, as do excessive heat or cold, we may begin to regain a state of balance by controlling our breath. We should strive to breathe slowly and deeply.

Our thoughts should be focused on productive outcomes, not those associated with the five emotive patterns. Most importantly, we should find time to listen to the messages that our bodies are sending.

Failing that, we pay the price in the form of illness and disease attacking our Three Treasures: Mind-Body-Spirit, the exclusive three-state connection.

Adrenaline cascade boosts our energy levels for fight or flight reaction

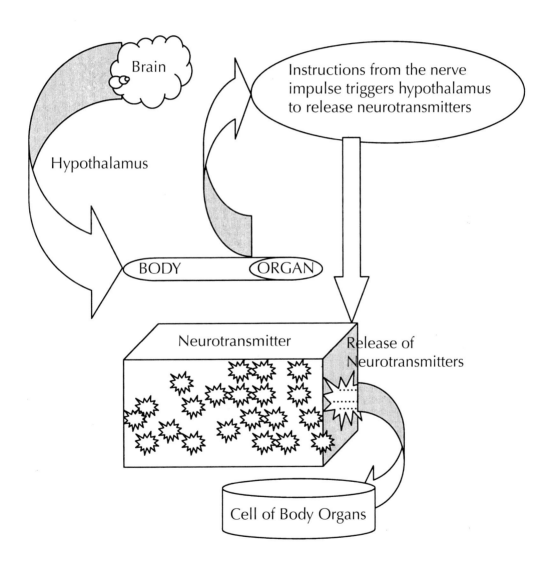

Stress Robs Your Three Treasures

THE SPIRIT-MIND-BODY CONNECTION is of multifaceted complexity and when optimally developed, leads to true oneness with inner symmetry and equilibrium.

Stress is a three-directional enemy. It will do harm in the form of:

1. Any type of condition that induces fear. (Spirit)
2. A disturbing environment. (Mind)
3. A disease. (Body)

Honest self-analysis and acknowledging that stress damages your health, are two critical steps in the process of taking the required measures to resist stress.

FIRST: Develop a process to identify situations which have caused you stress.

SECOND: Evaluate your own part and reaction to such stimuli in allowing the stress to become internalized.

THIRD: Determine how you reacted to stress.
   a) Reacted with anger?
   b) Another glass of wine?
   c) With vengeful thoughts?
   d) Blamed everything on someone else?
   e) Adopted the "poor-me" attitude?

This process of Identification, Recognition, Addressing and Remedial Action will provide a platform from which to prepare a daily schedule to regain your energetic balance and reduce Stress.

Spiritual stress has no connection with any religious dogma. Spiritual stress is best understood as one's spirit being low—the state in which a person is said to be dispirited. The individual must become alert to this invisible state of stress. When a person is unaware of stress and is therefore unable to manage this anomalous health hazard, unconscious stress will engender a deficiency of the Human Spirit. This is the meaning of spiritual stress. Moreover, any deficiency of spirit will result in a state of spiritual stress.

Listed below are examples of spiritually stressful ailments or conditions—some of which seem to accumulate, and subsequently deteriorate the health of the individual when improperly managed:

- A state of abject poverty
- Impending penury and enveloping torpor
- General boredom and ennui
- A lackadaisical attitude or disinclination
- Conditions of obesity and languor
- Health disinterest and antipathy
- The absence of motivation
- Self-loathing
- Having no intent to set objectives.
- An inability or reluctance to handle simple tasks
- Miscellaneous fear or trepidation of the unknown
- Media induced anxiety and fear
- Ubiquitous loss of self-reliance

Fortunately, the daily practice of Lion's Tail Qi Gong (ShiQi Qi Gong), which I will introduce shortly, will help you to cultivate sufficient quantity of Universal Qi. Universal Qi will then be converted to Spiritual Qi, because of your color-guided Qi meditative practice, thus enabling you to offset Stress.

Cultivated Spiritual Qi—when accumulated in sufficient quantities offers the practitioner, through his or her daily practice, some replacement of depleted inner energetic force. It will increase your endurance and fortitude and helps to prevent and hinder the progression of spiritual stress.

To say the least, the initial effort required to cultivate Spiritual Qi might at first seem strange. However, one must proceed with the task, especially if the individual is already under an attack of spiritual stress.

Such an individual should take heart and proceed with the stylized movement of Lion's Tail Qi Gong regardless of the stress being endured.

After beginning the practice of Lion's Tail Qi Gong, the symptoms of the condition or problem will at first be interrupted in their severity. Next, one will experience a reduction in the symptoms of stress. Later, the individual will begin to gain control of the effects of stress. With regular daily practice, one will develop the skills and ability to prevent the onset of stress itself.

A few of the stress-related ailments associated with the Mind-Body connection are the following:

- Suspect and/or restricted joints, irritable nerves, posture problems and frequent colds
- Increasingly protracted flu-type symptoms
- Abdominal pains and bloating
- Bouts of diarrhea, nutritional depletion, irritable bowel syndrome and migraines
- Skin complaints, hypertension and anxiety
- The stressed human system can also suffer from an assortment of physical problems, some similar to neck, shoulder and back pains. These aches or pains will appear to be random with possible unconnected twinges, perhaps even

Flow-chart

Showing the
developing Mental Stress
connection to a Physical Stress path.

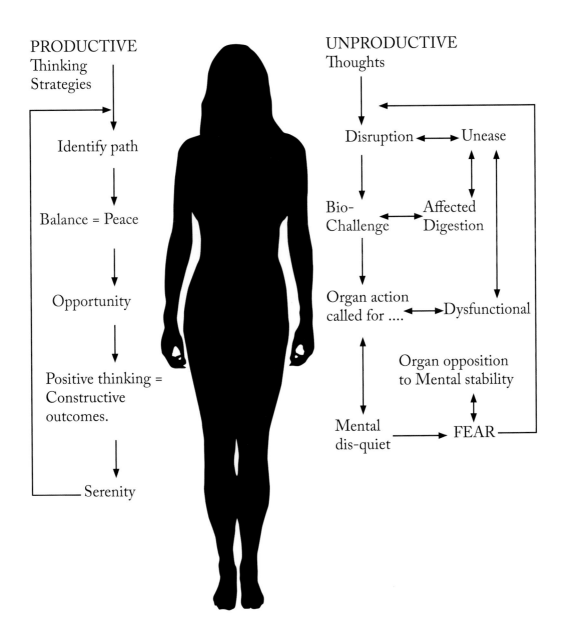

PRODUCTIVE
Thinking
Strategies

Identify path

Balance = Peace

Opportunity

Positive thinking =
Constructive
outcomes.

Serenity

UNPRODUCTIVE
Thoughts

Disruption ⟷ Unease

Bio-
Challenge ⟷ Affected
Digestion

Organ action
called for .... ⟷ Dysfunctional

Organ opposition
to Mental stability

Mental
dis-quiet ⟶ FEAR

intermittent headaches, or at other times, spontaneously discovered bone or muscular tension.

- Occasional anomalous aching of the bones of the spine
- Eating disorders, obesity, anger, hatred, envy, impatience, energetic deficiency and a host of other very disturbing signs and symptoms resulting from a compromised Mind-Body connection.
- On an emotional level, there could be periods of lack of sleep, intermittent loss of appetite and other persistent minor ailments.

The Stress-Disease Epidemic

ON THURSDAY APRIL 9, 2009, *The New York Times* published an article with a front-page sub-headliner entitled "Recession Anxiety Seeps Into Everyday Lives," reported by Pam Belluck.

The article discussed a woman who had neither lost her job nor her savings. She and her husband had always been conservative with their finances. But a few months earlier, she began having panic attacks about the economy, struggling to breathe and seeing vivid visions of "losing everything." In addition, she could not stop reading current economic reports.

The woman became so sick to her stomach that she lost twelve pounds and was unable to function. For the first time, at fifty-two years of age, she began psychotherapy and taking psychiatric medications.

The article discussed another stressed out woman who had routinely enjoyed eight hours sleep at night. Then, the stories of desperate clients flooding her employment service, began to jolt her awake at 2:00 A.M. Unable to return to sleep, she first began responding to emails, but that caused sleeping colleagues' BlackBerrys to wake them. Presently, during her attacks of insomnia, she studies business books and meticulously organizes her closets.

The article further reported, that with economic problems expected to continue for several months or years, experts observed that such reactions have become commonplace. Presently, anxiety, depression and stress are troubling people everywhere. Many have not suffered significant economic losses themselves, but worry they will, or simply react to pervasive uncertainty and media hysteria.

In London some years ago, more evidence was found of the increased broad-based acceptance of the dangers of stress in modern consciousness. The *Daily Mail* published an article entitled "Beating the Blues" (Sept. 10, 2005) in which the author reported, "One in five of the United Kingdom's population is reckoned to be suffering from stress." The report estimated, "apart from the human suffering, stress problems have cost businesses in excess of 3,700,000,000 English pounds sterling [\$7,067,000,000] per year." From the time this article was published, the cost of stress-related problems has skyrocketed each and every year. And there seems to be no let-up for the foreseeable future.

Another article published in the *Daily Mail,* claimed that at least 6.5 million working days are lost each year due to stress and its related complaints. The article made the emphatic statement that stress, apart from causing disease, accelerates the ageing process of all of our systems.

Apparently the National Health Service (NHS) of the United Kingdom has accepted and endorsed applied therapy for stress-related health problems within its workforce.

The immune system's behavioral interactions are at the very core of our health problems. Moreover, I am convinced that stress is the genesis of disease.

As noted earlier, stress has a varied gestation period. At times, it can be almost instantaneous, while in other instances, its effects can be protracted, taking years to produce the symptoms of disease on a physical or emotional level. Stress can quickly disable the immune system and thereafter attack us in our weakened constitution. When this occurs, the duration of our systems' dysfunction becomes prolonged.

Such health issues often appear to be unrelated, especially cases of previous stress-related ailments. This may be due to the fast attacking parameters of that particular stress condition. Then again, the effects may be demonstrated in a very long delay curve, occurring when the person is older. Or, the condition can be generated when a nutritional deficiency becomes intolerable, whereby the internal energetic defense processes have been severely weakened.

These types of conditions initiate changes at a molecular level that can cause a mutation to develop. At a cellular level, some individual cells will behave erratically. The person might feel somewhat uncomfortable, experience a state of uneasiness, but not be aware of the cause. With no identifiable signs and no apparent or visible symptoms, the sufferer will not be able to make the association. Therefore, there is nothing to call attention to a developing complaint. In most cases, internal conflicts and loss of energetic balance emerge after prolonged bouts of stress-induced problems. At one end of the health spectrum, a nervous breakdown may occur due to the absence of appropriate therapy and the unrecognized seriousness of the complaint.

The time for individuals to receive therapy or relief from stressful conditions can be long overdue. This delay may be due to the sufferer being unable to accurately identify the cause of and condition of the complaint. It can create an additional delay in receiving adequate or even the correct type of ministration. The person concerned will unknowingly be aiding and abetting the effects of stress.

By the time we know that we are ill, our immune systems would have already been subjected to severe and chronic pressures caused by stress.

These causes can be identified as acute and chronic.

1) ACUTE stressful factors include:
   Financial troubles, fear, family disharmony, noise, sleep disturbances, crowd activity, pedestrian and motorized traffic, isolation, hunger and severe temperature changes
2) CHRONIC stressful factors include:
   Vibratory parasitics, prolonged and/or serious illness, political and/or religious dogma, marriage or divorce, poverty, death, work issues and/or environment and media fear-mongering

Remember that stress is constant. It is accompanied by internal disturbances that can quell our worldly ambition and social inclinations. Stress is a part of our everyday existence and is in everything we do. Stress forms a significant part of every aspect of our society. It accompanies nearly all our experiences and will continue to grow and evolve as we do. It is an absolute fact of our lives of which we must remain aware.

It is we who must change to prevent its damaging effects.

More so now than ever before, our technological culture and society are geared towards stress as a way of life. Yet, in its very nature and at its core, stress is dysfunctional.

It is my sincere opinion that a spiritually defunct culture, regardless of any technological advancements, will be exposed to the problems associated with stress. In the midst of such a society or culture, a paroxysm not on a pathological platform, may not even produce noticeable symptoms.

As we become more technical and less spiritual, symptoms of stress that have arisen include, but are not limited to:

Anxiety, alcoholism, anger, crime, depression, eating disorders, heart disease, headaches, hypertension, obesity, sleep dysfunction, Type 2 diabetes and violent behavior.

Even more alarming is the fact that children are not immune to the problems caused by stress, and in some cases are affected more than adults. The United States populace suffers the ravages of stress from childhood onwards. A report by the American Academy of Pediatrics stated that in the year 2000 one in every five children in America had psychosocial problems that may well be stress-related.

On April 8, 2008, the *Daily Mail* published an article about administering bite-size GCSE (General Certificate of Secondary Education) standardized test to reduce the stress on students. The article looked at the effects of stress on teenaged pupils and the stress placed upon them by sitting for tests and examinations. The newspaper's education correspondent, Laura Clark, stated that teenagers would be allowed to retake parts of their GCSE tests in a more flexible manner. The testing board was concerned about the effects of previous methods of administering the exams regarding higher incidence of teenage stress. The proposed reforms were backed by the government watchdog agency, the Qualifications and Curriculum Authority.

Stress-induced dysfunctions in children and teens can include:

- Digestive upheaval
- Allergies
- Nutrient deficiency
- Intermittent loss of vitality
- Spasmodic colon
- Diagnosed cranial dysfunction
- Semi-permanent sinus problems
- Autonomic problems
- Urinary tract ailments
- Mechanical disorders
- Cases of impaired immune system
- Dental infections

Health complaints visible and prevalent on a national level might be due to the inherent stress factors within any such society whose path is without real spirituality and humanitarian endeavors.

It's a well-known fact that when more primitive societies modernize, the population is soon afflicted with what experts call "Western diseases": heart attacks, Type-two diabetes, and the other serious ailments previously discussed.

Another effect of stress and its neurogenic properties is the ever-present worldwide spread of obesity that results in chronic and fatal heart problems.

Stress creates depression, which may trigger alcoholism and/or insomnia. Also, the results of mental stress can initiate unnatural cognitive behavior. For example, journalists Lucy Cockcroft and Richard Edwards wrote an article for the *Daily Telegraph* (Jan. 11, 2008) headlined "Mother of twin girls kills herself just two weeks after their birth." The article described the mother as suffering from postpartum depression. A married woman, she stepped in front of a delivery van at dawn, two weeks after the birth of her twins, while her husband and babies slept.

Depression is a typical condition that new and expectant mothers are forced to bear. Sometimes they are perceived as being temperamental. At other times, they may be told that they are acting up or seeking attention, etc. They may be scolded for their depression and told they should behave and learn to cope like millions of other women.

I strongly contest this sort of disregard and misdiagnosis. Although new mothers are often highly emotional, the dismissive attitude toward any person's state of distress is cruel and short-sighted.

It is my sincere conviction that each human being has an individual biological reaction mechanism. This human mechanism is unique to each of us and forms the greatest part of our humanitarian and spiritual ethology. This same humanitarian and spiritual ethology is best displayed when we show great refinement, strength and concern for the higher, sacred things in life.

This innate ethology triggers our individual, unconscious stress response to the numerous traumatic situations that we are subjected to daily. This is how spiritual stress harms us at its most subtly invasive and definitely insidious line of attack. Stress has contributed, is currently contributing and will continue to contribute to an epidemic of aberrant behavior in developing and developed countries.

Evidently, some symptoms are viewed as being not directly connected or related to stress. Perhaps the ailment that the person is suffering from may not have been completely understood, given the numbers of patients that clinicians have to attend to.

In some cases:

a) The primary condition was not fully detected.
b) The cause of the complaint is anomalous.
c) There wasn't any family history of the malady.
d) The patient did not portray anything common to stress.
e) Stress was overlooked because of the type of illness.

However, in these circumstances, it does not mean that stress was not the common denominator.

There are many medicines which are prescribed to help alleviate some of the symptoms of stress. These allopathic treatments often cause deleterious side effects such as headaches and various pain-associated ailments.

Such drugs are provided by a number of flourishing pharmaceutical companies. They may actually help with reducing the nature of the complaint. But after some time, the effects of the drugs themselves may be worse than the original problem.

Pharmaceutical medications are directed to the symptoms, but not the root cause of the symptoms.

If the problem is not attended to directly, or the original cause is not universally accepted, then the complaint will not be accurately identified. Therefore, the treatment or therapy offered will be only palliative, addressing only apparently unconnected symptoms. Or, worse yet, addressing nothing whatsoever and causing dire side effects.

Here is an example of that possibility. In the *Daily Mail* (February 28, 2008), Jeremy Thomas, a former depressive, authored an article entitled "The Happy Pill Conspiracy." He wrote, "Drug companies put profit ahead of safety by failing to reveal evidence about their products," it has been claimed. "Psychiatrists have accused pharmaceutical companies of hiding unflattering data from drug regulators, GPs and the public."

The writer launched a withering attack on the ease with which the medical profession doles out "happy pills" pointing out that most of the 30,000,000 anti-depressants prescribed each year are useless. He quoted a landmark study by the University of Hull that showed widely-prescribed anti-depressants, such as Prozac, Seroaxt and Efexor work little better than placebos.

Thomas went on to write that much of the data on the effectiveness of anti-depressants was not fully publicized, thus people were being misled about the dire side effects such medications threaten. Suicidal ideation, anxiety, insomnia, headaches, nausea, and vomiting are just some of the problems created by taking these drugs. He quoted the policy of the Medicines and Healthcare Products Regulatory Agency, "it is a criminal offence for drug companies not to provide us with information about side-effects."

The article further states, "The news that antidepressants taken by tens of millions worldwide don't work is another step in the decline of what was a fantastically popular class of drugs."

The author further reported on the claims of the American Institute of Stress, "More than ninety per cent of all doctors' appointments have their origins in the mechanics of stress." The Institute reports that Americans consume more than five billion tranquilizers, millions of barbiturates, billions of amphetamines, and tons of aspirins every year.

These are conservative numbers and they are rising at a most frightening scale, with the inclusion of ever more dangerous drugs supplied daily and at an increasingly and alarming rate.

We must wake up!

Conditions of stress do not require pacification of the symptoms. They demand serious attention from all of us. The use of symptomatic camouflage only worsens and disguises the dire factors of spiritual deficiency.

Spiritual deficiency is the cause of our culture's continually escalating stress conditions. However, most people just want a magic pill, a happy pill to solve their health problems.

So they visit doctors who gladly write prescriptions for their patients. That's why the use of pharmaceuticals is at an all time high and increasing in volume day by day. Generally, manufacturers and dispensers of prescription and over-the-counter medications do not acknowledge your Three Treasures: Spirit, Mind and Body.

Our body's natural healing process is necessary first to trigger the immune system's response, thereafter enabling detoxification, and initializing enhancement by toning of the muscles, improving nourishment of the blood and strengthening the bones.

All of these, in addition to the process of kidney elimination of unwanted waste products, are interdependent functions. They form part of the wider internal system for good health.

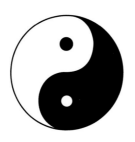

Part Two:
The Qi Gong Solution

The Search for Answers

Most of us search for answers to questions we hold within ourselves. Perhaps you are reading this book because you, like so many others, want to know:

- Why am I not feeling good?
- Why do I not look healthy?
- What is wrong with me?
- What direction should I take?
- Why am I stressed out all the time?
- What's gone wrong in my life?
- When will my fortune change for the better?
- What have I been doing wrong?
- Why me?
- Who can help me?

Typically, we look outside ourselves for answers on how to remedy pain, how to bring relief, change course, make atonement, correct failures, rectify costly errors, or fulfill our most pressing desires.

Perhaps we begin the search for something better, such as a better job, nicer friends, a bigger house, a more pleasing physique, and so on. We do this because we live in a world where organizations and individuals make money from us by promulgating the myth that more is better.

To achieve the goals they encourage, we turn to consultants and doctors. And in doing so, we become even more emotionally stressed.

The desire to find answers to our problems is so great and our need is so strong that the search becomes exhausting, like running on a treadmill—running, but not getting anywhere. In many cases, the search itself becomes the goal.

Yet, in reality we are merely squelching our desire and anesthetizing our pain, sometimes without even being aware of it. While doing this, we remember that somewhere, at some time, we heard that the answers to our questions lie within ourselves.

In a world of excess, the word "within" sounds like a stale cliché. The interior world has been relegated to a myth, a fabled cavern far away from anything realistic, recognizable or attainable.

Some physicians say that a pleasant pastime or hobby will take our minds off the daily stressful pressures. At one time, this actually may have had a ring of truth to it. But soon after, the pastime or hobby becomes competitive. When not fought against others, or media-driven self-image advertisements, then we struggle even against our very own selves and induce ever more stress.

However, we now know that there are various types of stress, and hence, different results are associated with each type of lifestyle pursuit. Pastimes and hobbies alone cannot ultimately prevent and reduce the levels of stress hormones. When hyper-anxious, one becomes unable to disperse stress-induced hormones. This is true even when engaged in regular exercise and attempts at relaxation.

In due course, such stress-related conditions will reach their maturity. This sets up the system for inflammatory responses. It is as if you were using rocket fuel to fill the gas tank of a small car whose engine is of minimum power capacity. Ultimately, the car's engine will burn out and interestingly, stressed people use the expression, "I'm burnt out."

Because stress hormones accumulate within our bodies, we must look at the type of help that will address that specific variety of stress.

Your quest for effective help requires independent thought, a re-examination of "the way things really are." You will need courage to approach current and future health issues differently than what our culture and society has set as the norm. The norm is a dependence-based culture, one that is financially and politically organized in an all-consuming and powerful ethos.

This culture has the ability to alter everything necessary to human happiness. It is designed to distort reality so as to achieve the ends of conglomerates of power who ever seek to control us—the unworthy masses, the "consumers." A great many individuals, who represent very powerful organizations, are most gainfully employed and vigorously engaged in seeking to manipulate our goals and thoughts.

To those so involved and financially concerned—whose intent should be to provide a modality that will make a reduction in the suffering of their clients/customers—I ask this one question: "For whom is this culture of dependency a good thing?"

A reliance on public health care and modern medical practices is anything but a good thing. It is risky, as my next disturbing piece of news reporting will indicate.

On January 23, 2008, a *Daily Express* headline blared, "£12,000,000,000 ($22,920,000,000) in NHS 'botch' fund." The article went on to reveal that opposition leaders had discovered that the National Health Service had set aside nearly £12 billion to pay compensation claims for flawed medical practices within the British public healthcare system. This money was earmarked to settle soaring lawsuits for bungled operations, superbug infections, incorrect diagnosis and other misfortunes suffered as a result of negligence.

The taxpayer-funded liability reserve was increased by £1.5 billion during the previous year. Tories warned that the huge sum was being concealed in the National Health Service accounts and would hamper government's ability to provide medical services (in this instance, perhaps it is a good thing)!

The article further stated "Last year the Clinical Negligence Scheme paid out more than 1 billion pounds. But trusts and hospitals only paid in £458 million, leaving a shortfall of £680 million. A Department of

Health spokeswoman is reported to have said, "The NHS Litigation Authority has rightly identified the £680 million net change within its accounts, as a deficit. These provisions represent liabilities that have yet to reach fruition, but which will fail to be paid in future years from scheme member contributions."

My concerns are for those who are suffering and being offered merely what has been endorsed and promoted as being the sole modality of any use, or the only one available. This treatment is only palliative. It does not achieve healing. While it is extended to those suffering from damaging health conditions, it comes nowhere near to treating the root causes of health conditions.

The customary phase exploited with indifference in reference to the serious emerging health situation we have been so diligent in identifying is, "Oh, it's only stress." The depth and invasive nature of stress at a molecular stage was not, and still is not fully appreciated by conventional health practitioners. With respect to providing real answers and solutions, a stalemate exists between those who are in, or approaching a state of chronic stress, and healthcare professionals.

However, the good news is that there are signs of a shift occurring in consciousness. Perhaps, it will become of sufficient magnitude to turn the tide of ill health that has been caused by a lack of awareness of the deleterious effects created by stress.

Some enlightened physicians and many forward-thinking individuals are now recognizing the dangers of stress and making the claim that stress is the number one cause of disease and illness.

After careful deliberation, I have decided to actively reveal information to those who are unaware of the underlying cause and effects of stress. And most importantly, I will offer solutions.

I intend to accomplish this task by offering this book. In addition, I will continue by any other means possible to spread the word and furnish such relevant information which may be of use to the general public. I shall continually strive to help as many people as possible to become aware of these ancient methods of conquering stress—ancient methods which have never been either more contemporary or of greater urgency.

The Way to cope, manage, reduce, prevent, and eliminate Stress is by the daily practice of Qi Gong—namely LAMAS Lion's Tail Qi Gong (ShiQi Qi Gong).

LAMAS Lion's Tail Qi Gong is easy to learn and will protect you against the invasive and destructive nature of "Perverse Qi."

Ancient Art Conquers Stress

IT IS INSPIRING TO DISCOVER how long some of the renowned practitioners of Traditional Chinese Medicine actually lived. They achieved what many of us want today—the ability to feel younger and live longer.

> CHANG SANG is said to have lived for 254 years.
> ZHANG DAO-LING lived 122 years.
> XU SUN lived 135 years.
> GE HONG lived 160 years.
> QIU CHU-JI lived for 189 years.

The list goes on and on and on.

Should any of these ages be even near the truth, one has to ask, "How did they do it?"

Their health secret is here revealed:

They practiced the Ancient Chinese meditation of Qi Gong.

In 1973 the Daoyin Silk Scroll, discovered at Mawangdui Hunan Province, Mainland China, was dated to be approximately 4,500 years old.

This discovery authenticated Qi Gong as *the* Ancient Chinese Healing Art, with the attendant philosophies that accompany the practice of Qi Gong. The Daoyin Silk Scroll depicts 44 human figures of different ages and both genders in different positions, practicing Qi Gong movements.

The practitioners' observations were centered on both the immediate and wider environment: including plants and trees covering various regions, the food that people consumed and the nature of their daily struggle for a menial existence.

The ancient sages also studied the characteristics and types of the local environment in which animals and fish dwelt. Particular emphasis during these observations was placed on the interaction of the immediate and extended environment and the health of the people therein.

The Qi Gong Masters also paid very special interest in the climatic variations of wind and water, the ebb and flow of the tides, the interplay between deep craters and tall mountains, the rise and fall of the sun, along with the waxing and waning of the moon.

These wise and spiritually knowledgeable ancients perfected a way to increase and enhance the quality and longevity of life, while abiding and living in harmony with planet Earth.

Currently, some stress management courses cover Action Orientated Instruction. Apparently, these offer an open confrontation with stress-related problems.

Such applications tend to alter or change one's perception of stress, while encouraging us to understand and modify our homes, immediate work spaces, recreation or leisure facilities, public community type environments and surrounding neighborhoods.

If we were privileged to see with the eyes of the ancients, we would begin to understand that such "modern conditions" as Sick Building Syndrome (see page 136), Seasonal Affective Disorder (sunlight absence disease), Cell Wall Degradation and other complaints—which have been referred to as newly discovered—were in fact being addressed by Qi Gong Masters thousands of years ago.

If we were to look through the eyes of ancient sages, we would recognize a series of old health-related issues that are now causing the widespread devastation, which we have observed in stress related illnesses.

These issues may seem to be apparently unconnected, but as we have discussed, they have their origins in stress. By adapting a natural and environmentally friendly approach to our daily lives, we would enjoy a longer, happier, and healthier lifestyle merely by protecting ourselves against stress.

Qi Gong masters from ancient times to the present day, view stress quite differently than anyone who has learned about health and the causes of illness and disease through conventional, modern methods.

The intention and input behind any holistic therapy and application is to treat the cause of the ailment. In the application of holistic methods, therapy is specifically for the spirit, mind and body agenda and not the apparent symptoms associated with the complaint.

Let me explain it this way: the internal movement of stress is what may be described as a continuously spiraling orbit. Without interruption, its path is that of a figure eight. It transfers itself into all areas of the host body and attacks on all three of our body domains.

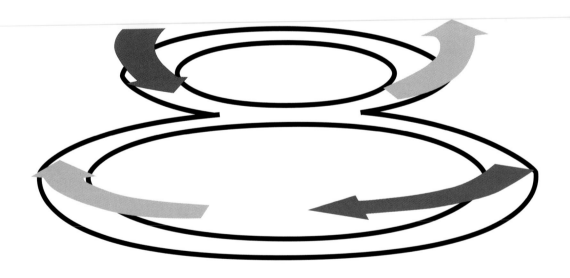

There are no start points from which the flow begins, nor are there any positions or points in any direction from which the flow may be imagined to end. The flow paths may be likened to the flux densities which circulate within the body.

The three body domains or Three Treasures—Spirit, Mind and Body—are governed by human biochemical electromagnetic fields. These internal "emotion generated fields" are not similar to the general electromagnetic fields that govern our physical world. These are emotionally produced bio fields with some very primitive means of inter-communication within the envelope; that is, within the body of the person concerned.

These bio-fields are completely different in that they propagate the continuously ever-changing multi-directional stress flow. To further understand how stress causes disease and illness, it is helpful to be generally familiar with the concept of Meridians in the Body.

The Theory of Meridians

THE MERIDIANS MAY BE THOUGHT OF as a network of pathways which conduct Qi into, around, and throughout the entire human system, providing Qi to specific organs within our bodies.

Each of the Twelve Major Meridians or Channels form pathways of communication and transportation.

The other Eight Major Meridians are referred to the Eight Extraordinary Vessels and are in reality storage devices for Qi.

Qi reserves held within these Eight Extraordinary Vessels are there to nourish the five pairs of Yin Yang Organs, that are accepted by Oriental medicine. These Eight Extraordinary Vessels also assist in the circulation and movement of smooth Qi within the body where desirable, such as in the transmission of Intentional Qi. It is said that the transmission of Intentional Qi may be directed only by a highly skilled Qi Gong intuitive healer.

Whenever there is a deficiency in Qi, the Eight Extraordinary Vessels will attempt to make up for the Qi deficiency.

These reservoirs of Qi can be accessed and enabled to provide Qi reserves. They can be engaged by the use of some specific Qi cavities (nebulous holes) which are connected to the Eight Extraordinary Vessels. (The Meridians and Extraordinary Vessels are referred to as Channels only when they are engaged.)

When the enabled actions of Qi Cavity connections are performed, they function as exclusive pathways or gates which open or close the Meridians when switched on by the use of human bio-chemically produced electromagnetic lines of force. Hence, they provide pathways to connect to the Qi reservoirs.

The gates are used to adjust the strength and smoothness of Qi flow between the Twelve Meridians or Channels (similar to rivers) and the Eight Extraordinary Vessels or Channels (reservoirs).

At various periods throughout one's life, whenever it becomes necessary, the Qi reservoirs or storage vessels can and will release Qi on demand. Qi will also release itself whenever it senses the need, especially in the case of hypostasis (the suppression of a gene by the effect of an unrelated gene).

When a person has suffered a traumatic experience, or has been subjected to some form of stress, be it at a Spiritual, Mental or Physical level, the Qi in some of the main channels will immediately become deficient.

A stressful experience will cause particular organs to be correspondingly subjected to pressure and additional forms of stress. Qi then rapidly accumulates around those organs. As soon as this occurs, the reservoirs must release more Qi to supplement the deficiency and increases Qi circulation to prevent any additional damage.

If the reservoir is unable to do so, stress enters a chronic stage and disease will attack the system in the guise of Perverse Qi. Perverse Qi is very harmful, invasive and the most disruptive energetic causative substance or agent that attacks the host body. It first disables the host, then eventually destroys it.

The main point of consideration is that the Chinese Medical Meridian system is an energetic distribution network which continually oscillates throughout the curvilinear physical and energetic flux densities.

This concept is completely dissimilar to the conventional Western medical view of the human internal systems. Hence, a traditional Chinese practitioner treats complaints in a way that is entirely different from the conventional Western medical practitioner. Having said that, many millions of people have heard of acupuncture, a Chinese modality that works with the Meridians. Though it was once outlawed, it is now used extensively in conventional and mainstream medical practices.

In a Metro Health article titled "Finer Points of Medicine" (Feb. 25, 2008), reporter Lisa Scott wrote, "Research released this month by the University of Maryland says women who have acupuncture while undergoing IVF (*in vitro* fertilization) treatment have a 65 per cent increased chance of getting pregnant."

Scott also reports that acupuncture was found more effective than conventional medicine in treating back pain. (In Great Britain, back pain is the primary complaint of workers taking sick days.)

In the article, she explains acupuncture by discussing "Qi flow along the internal twenty-one Meridians/Channels/Vessels, twelve Regular Meridians, Eight Extraordinary Vessels and extra channel from the Spleen." She states that acupuncturists can help the patient's body heal itself by encouraging the production of endorphins that stimulate the immune system.

The article quotes Dr. Mike Cummings, the director of the British Medical Acupuncture Society (BMAS) who informs us that the society has trained nearly 5,000 doctors in this ancient art. He also points out that acupuncture has gradually been accepted into mainstream Western medicine. It has proven successful in treating insomnia and decreases anxiety among recovering drug addicts by increasing melatonin levels. In addition, acupuncture has demonstrated significant value in improving energy levels in patients undergoing chemotherapy treatments.

Acupuncture was once called "Hot Needle" in China. Prior to that, it was a part of the practice of Qi Gong healing culture and has been used as a healing modality by Qi Masters for thousands of years.

In the past, Qi healers used their index fingers (not needles) to stimulate the body's healing responses and thereafter to offer resistance to "Perverse Qi." By using Intentional Qi, Qi healers were able to force Perverse Qi to leave the body's Regular Meridians. This is particularly useful in preventing the onset of stress, which—as we have been at pains to demonstrate, is the origin of disease.

Stress can affect the entire nervous system, causing varied and seemingly unconnected chronic health problems, some of which may become disabling. Mental stress is one of a series of conditions that we all—each and every one of us, have experienced or will experience at some point during our lifetimes. This sort of stress has neither boundaries nor limits. It may even enter your system under the guise and pretext of exhilaration.

Regardless of your personal circumstances, you will have to come to terms with the reality that stress is inevitable unless you practice some form of stress prevention technique. Stress first begins at a mental level. Thereafter, it will develop and attain full maturity evolving into disease.

Practicing Qi Gong, and following the other suggestions offered in this book, will help the Spirit-Mind-Body connection to offer resistance to attacks of stress. The techniques I am sharing here also provide the reader with opportunities to heal from within. Qi Gong encourages smooth Qi flow, and smooth Qi flow is the key to radiant health. Herein is your key to good health and the prevention of illness.

I am providing extensive information and disciplines, allowing you to choose that which suits you best. I also recommend a gradual and focused shift away from the pharmaceuticals and potions that are available with and without prescriptions. Complementary and holistic sources offer completely different and often varying solutions to the numerous effects of stressful conditions. These solutions might be as far apart as chalk and cheese with respect to conventional medical approaches.

Because we are a spiritually free people, you will have to make a choice. Herein, we are offering information that completely departs from common Western allopathic treatment options. You need to choose the particular culture or philosophy that you feel will be the most dynamic in the production of positive results for your personal health.

I earnestly believe Qi Gong is the ultimate solution to stress-generated disorders within the human system. Because of the body's energetic distribution network, every prescription and non-prescription medication will have unpleasant and in some cases very chronic side effects.

However, there are no unpleasant or discordant side effects from the practice of Qi Gong.

While conventional medical practitioners accept that the veins, arteries, blood vessels and capillaries carry blood around the body, they have yet to come to terms with the concept that Qi permeates everything within the universe.

Within a living human organism, Qi travels along the Meridians/Channels/Pathways.

Just because people cannot see Qi, it does not mean that Qi is not real. We also cannot observe wind or electricity, but know that they exist.

Here is my suggestion. Make the effort to engage in serious reflection and take a look at your own beliefs. Re-examine some of your previous thoughts, actions and the decisions you have made in the past. Only then will it become possible for you to be awakened to the consciousness, opinions, feelings and beliefs of others who may hold the possibility of truth for you.

Qi Gong deals with forces and feelings that many in Western culture neither experience or accept. Some of the nay-sayers are highly educated people who perceive the world in a more limited manner. My guess is that since you are seeking answers in this book, you are not entirely satisfied with their vision of the world. So let us do some reflecting together on the nature of subjective experience.

Take body temperature as an example:

Suppose you are experiencing a very high temperature that was not caused by your environment, nor initiated by the weather.

We are considering a feeling of excessive body heat that has not been artificially induced, but that you can feel wherever you may be.

It is reasonable to assume that you alone feel this temperature increase within yourself. And, if you are the only one sensing the heat, then the question becomes whether or not the heat really exists.

If someone touches you and also feels it, then it may be accepted that this condition apparently does exist.

On the other hand, if no one touches you, or no one uses any type of device or equipment to measure your temperature, but you still feel extreme heat, does it mean that you are not experiencing a high temperature?

In other words, are your feelings and thoughts dependent on achieving consensus? If that is the case, you may have a difficult time discovering reality. For example, it may be possible that no one will agree with you regarding your personal experience of a high temperature. But just because others have no experience of your condition, does not mean that you are not feeling warm!

Does this imply that your experience is purely in your mind, a mere figment of your imagination? It doesn't matter because you are actually experiencing a condition that confirms your personal reality.

Think of the practice of Qi Gong in the light of this example. I encourage you to make the effort (if only as an experiment at first), to practice the techniques that you will discover in this book. If you do, you will find yourself on the path of self-healing. You will begin feeling better, become increasingly energized, more alive, healthier, happier and more stress-free. At that time, you can decide whether or not such feelings of well being are actually real! My ancestors and I, as well LAMAS Qi Gong Masters, various Qi Gong instructors, other practitioners and students over the millennia—proclaim that Qi Gong is an effective means of self-healing and enjoying a high quality, spiritually-awakened life for you and your loved ones.

Take Control of Your Health with Qi Gong

Su Wu was an esoteric Grandmaster of Qi Gong. It is believed he lived between 140 B.C. and 60 B.C. Ssu ma Chien, known as the "Grand Historian of China," is one of many scholars who refer to Su Wu as a man of letters and a powerful military leader. He earned his legendary status as a warrior with amazing physical dexterity, endurance and faithfulness against a challenging and skillful enemy.

Letters sent by General Li Ling to Su Wu following his release from prison praised Su Wu's physical skills, bravery and fortitude. Su Wu's ability to survive nearly twenty years of imprisonment and his other feats are attributed to his practice of the once esoteric art of Qi Gong.

Qi Gong is the ultimate of all Chinese Healing Arts, the ancient and original one.

Qi Gong calms the mind, rejuvenating and replenishing the body, while awakening the spirit.

Qi Gong is discreetly powerful. It prevents stress, strengthens the immune system, while also improving the endocrine, respiratory, circulatory and digestive systems.

Qi in this context is NOT translated to mean "True Qi" or life force." But it is to be considered the by-product that is produced by the practice of Qi Gong and the resultant flux, commonly known as energy.

Gong translates as "acquired skill or ability." In some instances, Gong can also mean the opening and or closing of the internal gates. These are specific areas within the body's internal organic machinery, which includes the cauldron. The cauldron is situated within our gravitational center, three 'cun' below the site of the umbilical cord. (One cun is the distance between any one knuckle of one finger and another knuckle of the same finger on the same hand.) The cauldron is the area in which our food, along with Oxygen, physical movement, individual thoughts, and the human internal bio-chemical environs are combined to produce the true life force known as Qi.

This description of Qi is not to be confused with cultivated Qi. Cultivated Qi is manifest or discernible through the practice of Qi Gong.

Qi Gong is a mental and physical discipline involving breathing techniques accompanied by movement and discrete visualization. These breathing techniques will develop a persona of relaxed and peaceful mentality. When combined with disciplined meditative movement, the practice will repair and strengthen the human physical and immune systems. Qi Gong color-guided Visualization gently leads the practitioner to the quiet place within the self.

The primary objective of Qi Gong practice is to enable the purging of any toxic emotional residues from within the body tissues. This prevents the possibility of stress-producing energetic stagnation.

A strengthening and balancing of our internal and external bio-energetic fields will produce the desired outcome. Hence, stress is reduced and a sense of well-being and serenity will be achieved.

Effective help can be sought from those knowledgeable persons whose intent is to provide a modality for the reduction of stress at any level.

It takes an external view by an unbiased observer to perceive and reveal the direction needed to improve health—a direction that will produce the best and very dynamic results.

Better self-monitoring and trying to understand your own health needs are vital. However, the practice of looking at one's health is a task commonly avoided by most people. Yet, conscious attention such as this is vital to the prevention and/or control of problems in their early stages.

If you are unable or reluctant to do this for yourself, please contact a reputable Qi Gong Master practitioner. He or she should be willing to help you address your health situation.

First, obtain details of someone who has a good Qi healing reputation. If such a person is unavailable in your immediate area, find out where and by whom you can obtain meaningful assistance. (I have provided a contact list of my associates in the appendices.)

Without accurate information about stress problems, it is very difficult to either provide or obtain the best advice on personal practices, medicine, or therapy that may be available.

Find a knowledgeable Qi Gong Master practitioner, and begin learning how to take control of your own health. Taking charge of your health is a necessary first step to avoiding and preventing future punitive attacks of stress.

Here are two ways to avoid and prevent the damages of stress:

1. Participate in a course of transmitted Meditative Qi healing sessions to reduce the transient cavitations (disturbances of body fluids caused by holes which mimic Qi cavities). Such transient cavitations can act as a restriction to smooth Qi flow.
2. Learn from a true Qi Gong Master, and then practice on daily basis, a Qi Gong stress-reducing meditation daily with synchronized movement and enhanced visualization techniques.

The implementation of these techniques on a daily basis will allow your system to heal. The goal of daily practice of Qi Gong is the achievement of a homeostatic state of well being and true inner balance. Only then will you finally enjoy a happier lifestyle.

Breathing is the key. This fact was underlined in an article the *Daily Mail* (May 3, 2008) entitled "Stress Out?" The article stated, "If you think listening to a Gregorian chant is relaxing, singing it could be even better. The regular breathing it demands, along with the musical structure, can melt away stress, researchers claim." It also discussed the work of Neuroscience lecturer Alan Watkins from Imperial College in London. Watkins heads a company that helps executives work well under stress. He asserts that learning how to control breathing can help improve one's emotional state. He discussed a recent study, in which five monks had their heart rates and blood pressure measured over a 24 hour period. "In a day that included the hardly stressful practices of quiet contemplation, prayer, and scripture study, their heart rates and blood pressure still dipped to their lowest points when chanting."

The development of respiratory power and control is fundamental to successful Qi Gong training. The breathing pattern must be quiet, long, deep, soft and even, for the mind to become peaceful and calm.

Therefore, in order to regulate the mind, one must first master the regulation of one's breath.

I call this Disciplined, Controlled, Respiratory Movement (DCRM) (the term is my own). With daily practice, such disciplined, controlled respiratory movement (DCRM) will generate and produce within you an aerobic type internal action that improves cardiovascular performance, as well as an overall level of fitness.

The series of physical movements performed during Qi Gong practice is called Daoyin (leading and guiding the cultivated Qi). Such movements are all done in a synchronized and sustained controlled manner, in harmony with slow deep breaths.

In Chinese philosophy, there is a direct correlation between breath and emotion.

Any excess in emotion leads to an irregular breathing pattern.

This negative process results in the body becoming stressed, and stress causes the breakdown of health.

A very important secondary improvement produced by Qi Gong is in the post-movement "feel good" sensation. This "feel good" factor is achieved without the physical and mental stresses generated by many recreational activities and sports.

Qi Gong encourages the brain to secrete serotonin, a vital cerebral fluid. This is a very much needed natural chemical that opposes the attacks of "Perverse Qi"—those energies whose origins are responsible for and accompany the onset of stress.

Qi Gong addresses the essence of a person, the Spirit-Mind-Body connection.

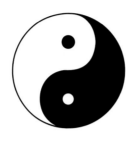

Part Three:

Qi Gong Tools
to Health and Happiness

Activity: Breathing Color

Because of our fast-paced society, within various stages of our worldly existence, our thoughts are constantly centered upon the means of survival and the acquisition of various artifacts. During periods of this type of mental activity, our breathing becomes shallow. It is therefore much less productive for longevity, especially if we had never sought to learn how to focus on our life force. When this trend of shallow breathing begins to approach a critical point, our bodies quickly come under the pressures of internal bio-chemical changes and develop what we have been referring to as stressful conditions.

Such bio-chemical changes and their developing stressful conditions invade the cells of our organs, because their beginnings are of a cellular nature. Such emotional and bio-chemical changes may be viewed as molecular disturbances, destroying our spiritual, mental, and physical equilibrium.

To counteract this state of non-equilibrium, one should begin to cultivate Qi.

Set aside a time with no interruptions from phones, computers, all manners of electronic or electromotive devices and from people who do not share a similar health-regenerative intent.

This is your period of complete cerebral cortex excitation suppression. It is time to allow the parameters of your brain to be at rest for rejuvenation.

Qi Gong movement (Daoyin) can be done sitting, standing, or lying down. However, for reasons related to metabolism and oxygen, a standing position is best.

Place the tip of your tongue gently between your front teeth and the gum line of your upper jaw. Your mouth remains closed at all times. Breathe quietly through your nostrils. Choose one colored circle that gives you the most relaxing and peaceful frame of mind. Close your

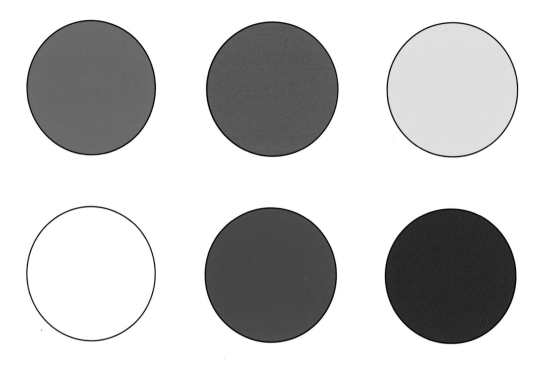

eyes. Visualize the shape and color of the Circle that you have selected for your Qi Gong visualization. Relax, close your eyes, and breathe very slowly and deeply. Let your mind be at peace. Continue for five to ten minutes before starting to practice your LAMAS Lion's Tail Qi Gong.

Visualization requires the mind to focus, and has been shown to produce various beneficial results. When we engage in the use of chosen or desired colors, we are employing the bio-intermodular products that are enhanced by the very positive sub-harmonic energies of the individual concerned. The preventative modality of Qi Gong, that is, the procedure of calming your mind and the benefits of focusing your thoughts on positive and meaningful outcomes, will actively contribute to smooth Qi flow.

Lion's Tail: A New Chapter of Your Life

Presented here are the instructions you have waited for as we patiently and painfully outlined the problems facing modern society.

Now you can start a new chapter that will serve you for the rest of your life. You can finally begin preventing the damages of stress with Lion's Tail (ShiQi) Qi Gong.

What was once esoteric family knowledge, Lion's Tail Qi Gong was practiced in Guyuan, a province of Ningxia, in the Mainland of China during the Qin Dynasty of the third century B.C. Lion's Tail is the only Qi Gong form created and developed specifically to reduce the stress already within the human bio-system. Lion's Tail is designed to prevent the damaging effects of stress and eventually, to eliminate stress.

Lion's Tail Qi Gong (ShiQi Qi Gong) also cultivates Prenatal Qi.

There are five main aspects of Qi Gong practice:

a) Controlled Meditation
b) Respiratory Regulation
c) Dynamic Visualization
d) Disciplined Breathing
e) Movement Synchronized with Breath

These are the five distinct parts that when combined, will aid the practitioner to fully realize his or her own personal objectives.

Meditation and movement, when practiced together within the program taught by Lion's Tail Qi Gong, allow you to find your center and to sense the effects of Qi circulating throughout your body. Meditation and movement are two discrete components. When combined,

Day	Minutes	Before practice sensations experienced	After practice
Mon.			
Tues.			
Wed.			
Thurs.			
Fri.			
Sat.			
Sun.			

they provide a completely different experience than either meditation on its own, or movement on its own.

To begin, it is essential to maintain a good posture during meditation. At first, this might feel uncomfortable, but one must persevere and not give in to distractions or disruptive influences.

Part of the process of meditation is the centering of oneself.

Each and every sensed impression or experienced sensation should be viewed as rungs on a ladder. It is only by using each rung, and moving step by step, that we can aspire to the state of no mental or physical distraction.

DISCIPLINED CONTROLLED RESPIRATORY MOVEMENT (DCRM).

DCRM is a Qi Gong principle that provides overall health improvement to the Qi Gong practitioner. When movement, meditation and visualization are combined, we approach the point of using DCRM as the foundation of our stress prevention routine.

Ancient Qi Gong practice is a form of moving meditation.

Your practice should be done on a daily basis. Regular work with Qi Gong will help you to adopt a moderate and healthy lifestyle. You will then be well on your way to conquering the harmful effects of stress in your daily environment, as well as healing yourself from the deleterious effects created by stressful conditions before you began the Lion's Tail practice.

Once they are alleviated, people tend to forget the magnitude of their complaints! Make several copies of this chart to record your sessions and reactions. This will also help you to appreciate the value of Qi Gong practice in your daily life and enhance your resolve to continue. When you are finished each day, write in a diary or use the chart provided on the opposite page to document your progress.

Here are some additional suggestions to consider before you begin. In the following pages, I am providing a series of photographs of the sequence of Lion's Tail (ShiQi Qi Gong) stylized postures and breathing techniques. Below each photo, are written instructions to help to help guide you in the proper breathing and motion. You may read and follow the instructions as provided here. We have purposely used a quality sewn binding process for this manual so that you can open and lay the book flat without damaging it.

Please also take advantage of the full-color wall chart we have included with this book to help with your practice.

There are also other practices you can do to help you learn and memorize the Lion's Tail instructions.

1) Writing down the instructions will help you to memorize and better understand them.
2) I have produced a DVD entitled *Lion's Tail Qi Gong* that will help make the simple instructions even clearer should the need arise, and show you how I do the practice. Contact information for ordering is provided at the end of this book.
3) You can also make an audio recording of the instructions using your own voice by reading them into a tape recorder and playing it back while doing the practice.

Other details to remember about Qi Gong and the meaning of the instructions include the following ideas:

1) Remember that one inhalation and one exhalation are equal to one breath.
2) Usually, when your arms change direction, you change from inhaling to exhaling or vice versa.
3) Qi Gong harmonizes spirit, mind, and body with the movement of limbs and your breathing acting as one entity.
4) All Qi Gong breathing and movements are done smoothly, slowly and gently.

If at first you need to take an extra breath, do so. It is OK. You are in a learning process.

Once you've memorized the movements and breaths, you'll enjoy them more, but for now, you're still learning. Most importantly, don't get stressed during the learning process!

Here are some more helpful tips for success in Lion's Tail Qi Gong.

a) If you have problems that will distract you from your practice, resolve to solve them tomorrow.

b) It is best not to eat for at least an hour before practice. You should drink only water thirty minutes before you start.

c) Practice must be in a warm and safe environment.

d) Wear comfortable clothing and footwear.

e) Subdued, soft music is acceptable if it helps you to relax.

f) Turn off cellular and landline phones.

g) Prohibit all other interruptions.

h) To avoid the onset of stress, try to practice on a daily basis for a minimum of fifteen minutes. However, ideally, Lion's Tail Qi Gong would provide dynamic and maximum results when a practice period is done for at least thirty minutes each day.

Daily practice will protect you from the harmful stages of stress and its life threatening effects. As you continue, your daily practice will also provide recuperative healing.

After practice, you will experience a reduction in your sense of stress.

The suggested requirement is daily practice and the adoption of a moderate, healthy life style.

OK, you are now about to improve your health.

Gently place the tip of your tongue between the gum line and front teeth of your upper jaw, that is at the top of your mouth.

Your lips should remain softly closed throughout the entire movement.

Breathe very quietly via the nostrils. It is unnecessary to make any sounds.

The following series of pictures demonstrate the movements of Lion's Tail Qi Gong. The Chinese name for this ancient wisdom of Qi Gong practice is ShiQi Qi Gong.

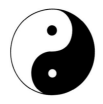

Grandmaster Lowe Demonstrates
Lion's Tail Qi Gong Postures
ShiQi Qi Gong

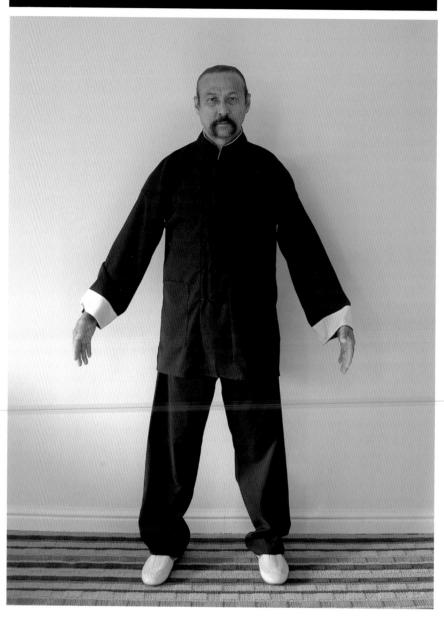

Relax, do not move, take nine slow deep breaths, relax.

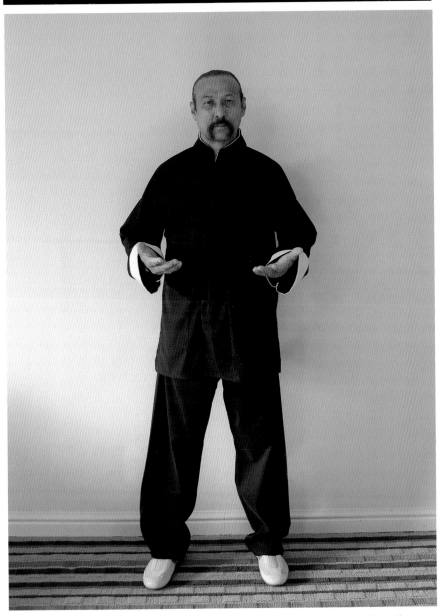

Inhaling slowly, raise both of your hands until they reach the chest sternum area.

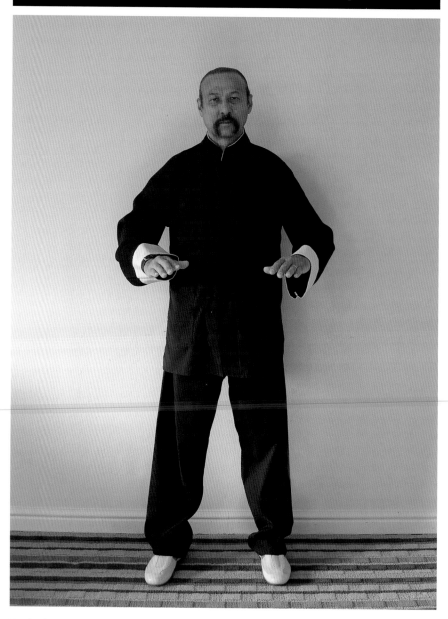

Exhaling, very slowly rotate palms to face downward.

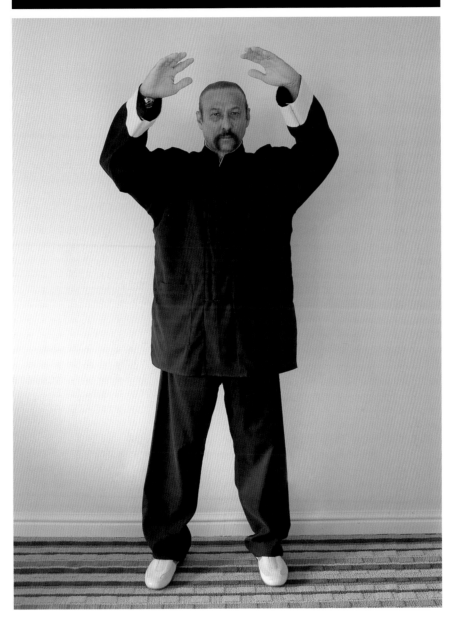

Inhaling, slowly as you begin to raise both of your hands until hands are level with top of head.

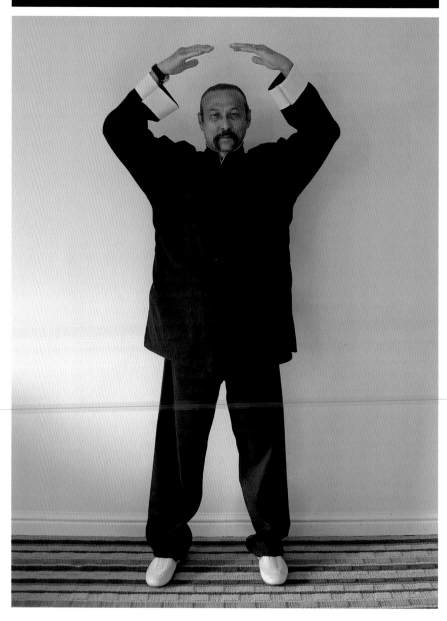

Exhaling, raise hands until overhead.

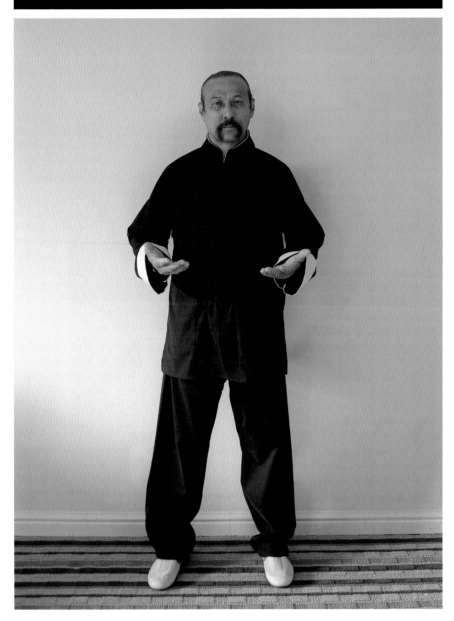

Inhale slowly, lower arms to chest.

Exhale slowly, rotate palms to face upward.

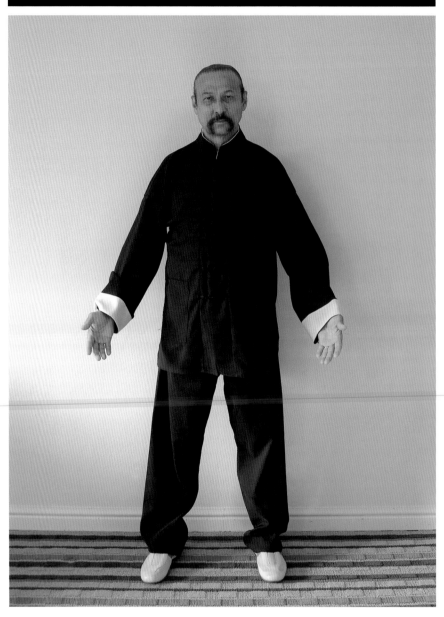

Exhaling lower hands.

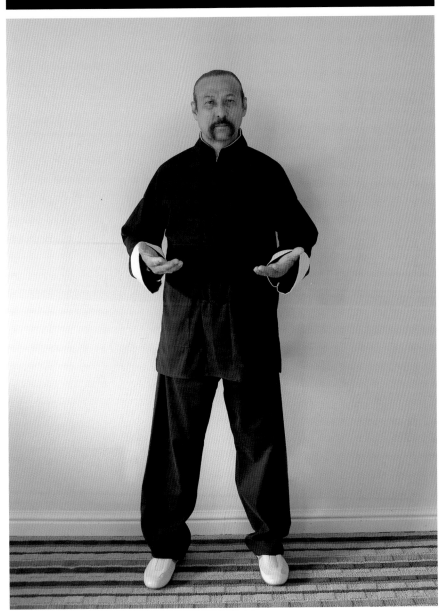

Inhaling slowly, raise arms until level with sternum as shown.

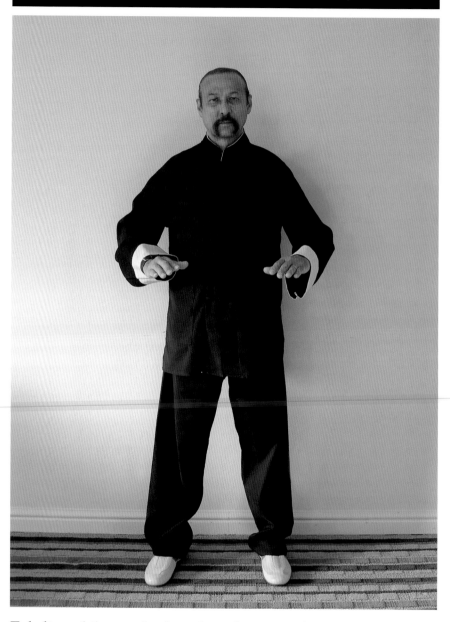

Exhaling while very slowly and gently rotating both of your hands until the palms are facing downward.

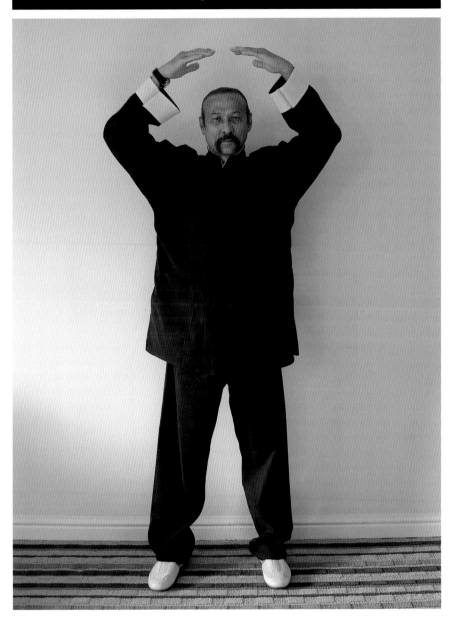

Exhale completely, raise hands over head.

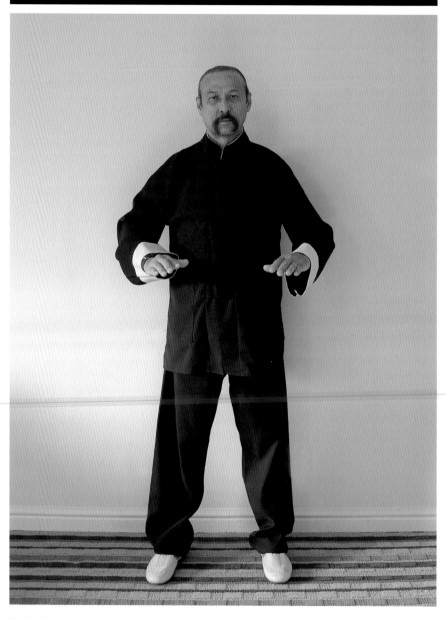

Inhaling while you commence lowering hands until they are level with your chest.

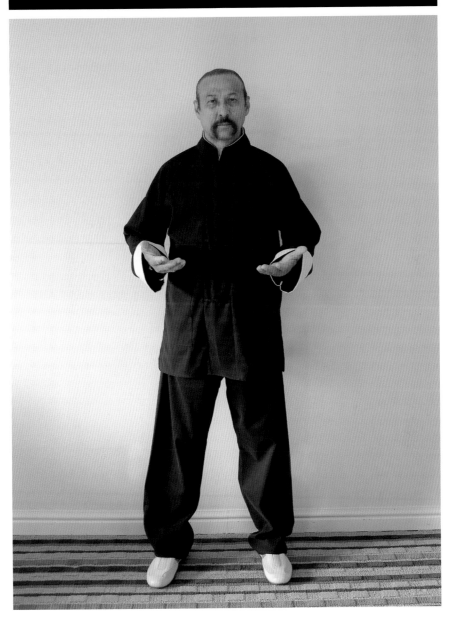

Exhaling rotate both hands as above.

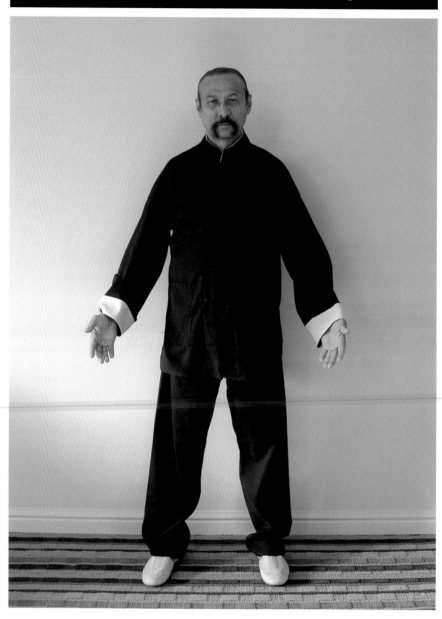

Exhaling lower hands.

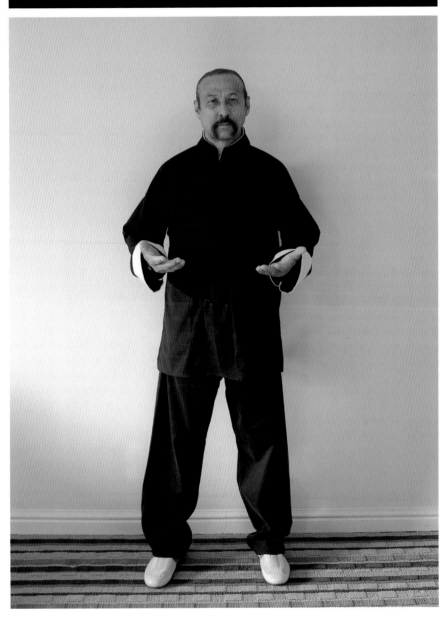

Inhaling, raise both hands as above.

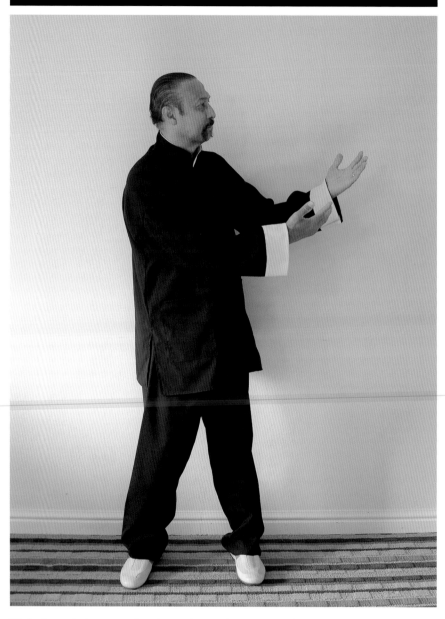

Exhale, while very slowly and gently moving both hands to your left.

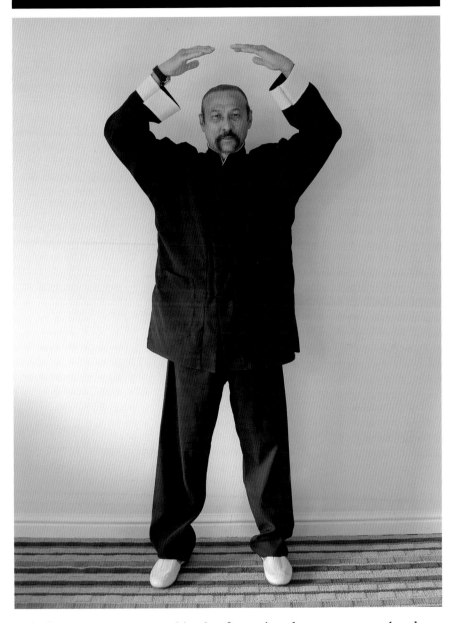

Inhale, moving arms until both of your hands are over your head, palms facing downward.

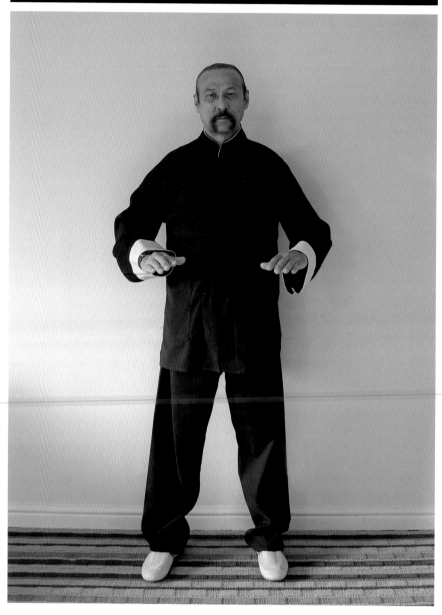

Exhaling very slowly lowering arms to chest/sternum level with palms facing downward.

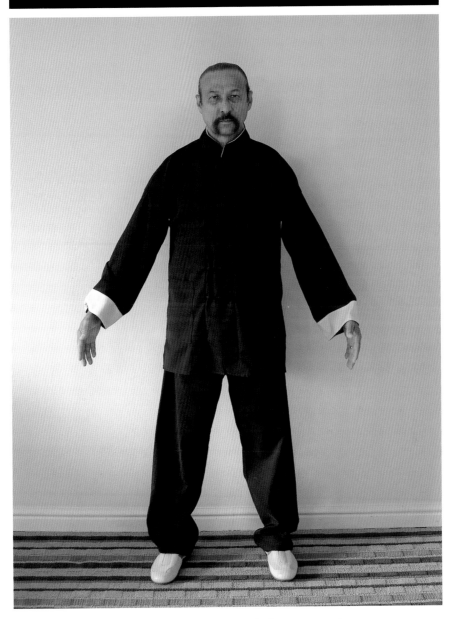

Exhale gently lowering both arms until they are as shown.

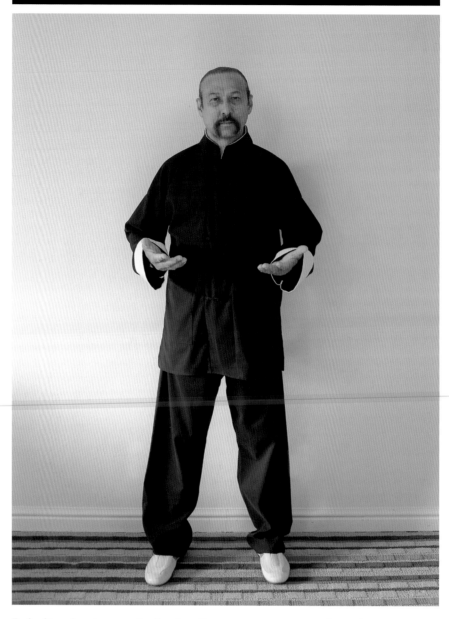

Inhaling begin to raise both of your arms to your chest / sternum level.

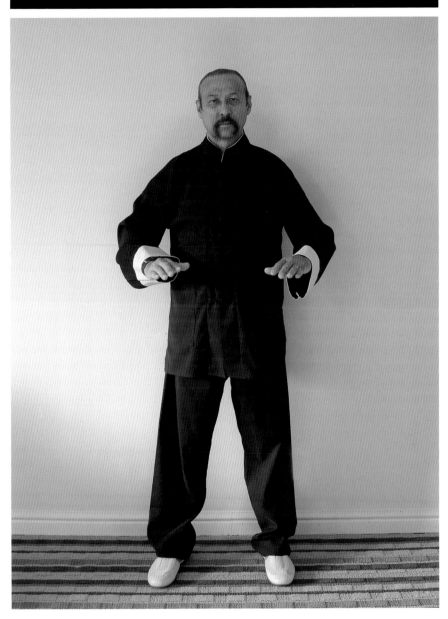

Exhaling rotate both hands.

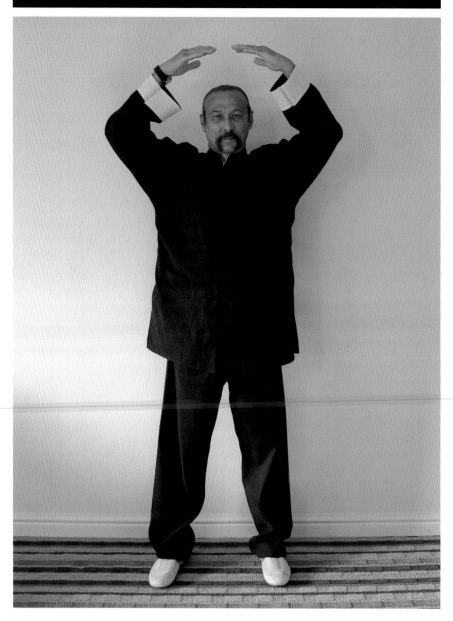

Inhale, as you begin to move both hands to the top of your head.

Exhaling as your hands go to the position as above.

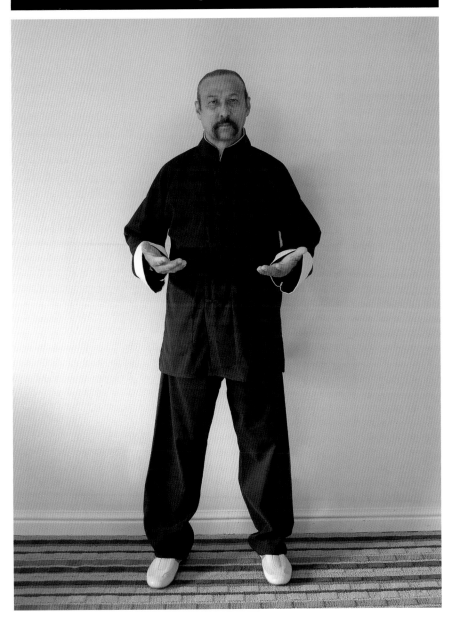

Inhaling lower arms to sternum, then exhale and rotate both palms to face upward.

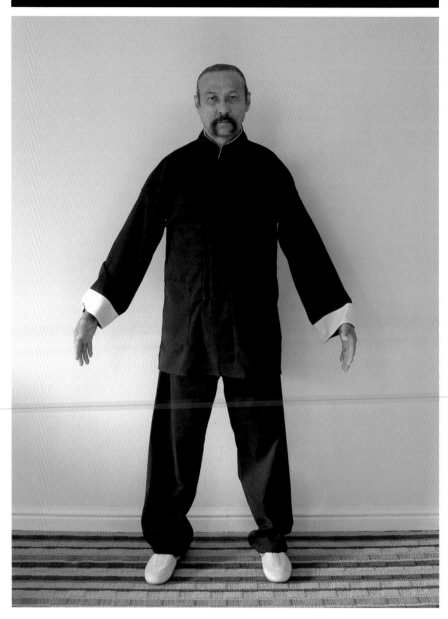

Exhale completely while lowering hands.

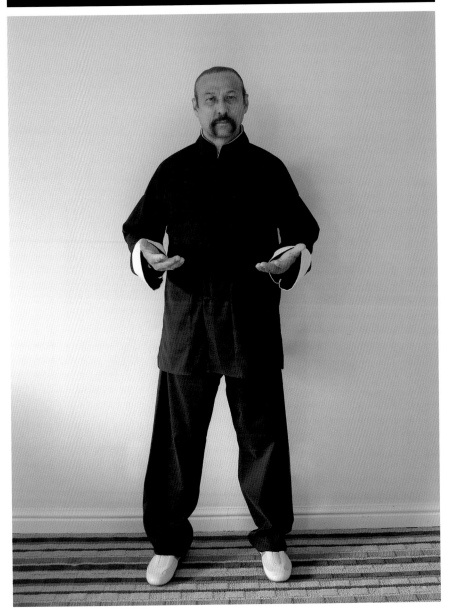

Inhale slowly raise arms to sternum.

Exhaling slowly rotate palms to face upward as shown.

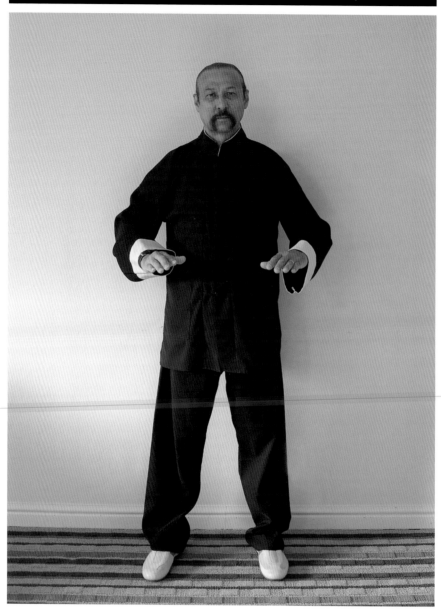

Exhaling rotate both hands.

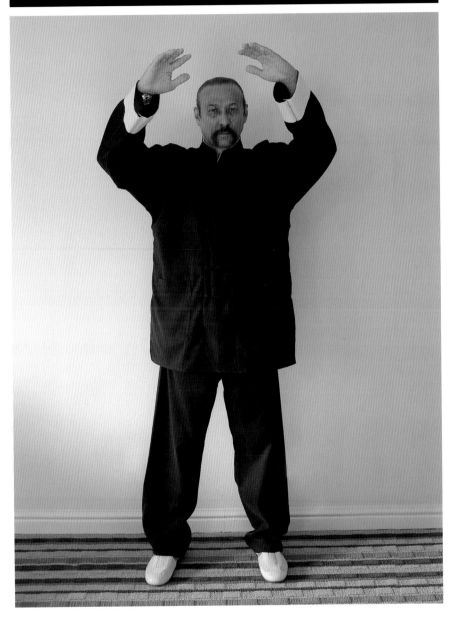

Inhaling, gradually raise both arms head high.

Exhale, and move your hands as above.

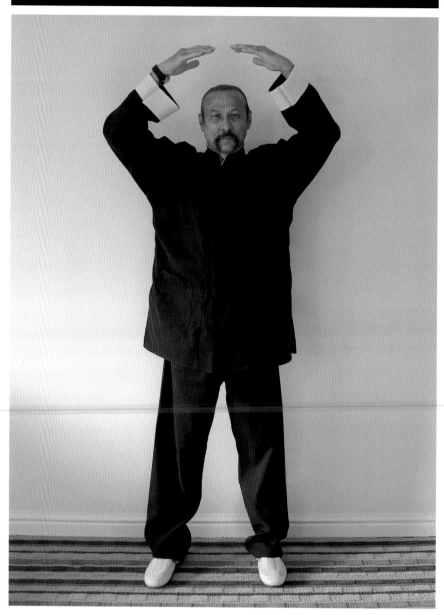

Exhaling slowly raise both arms until palms are over your head.

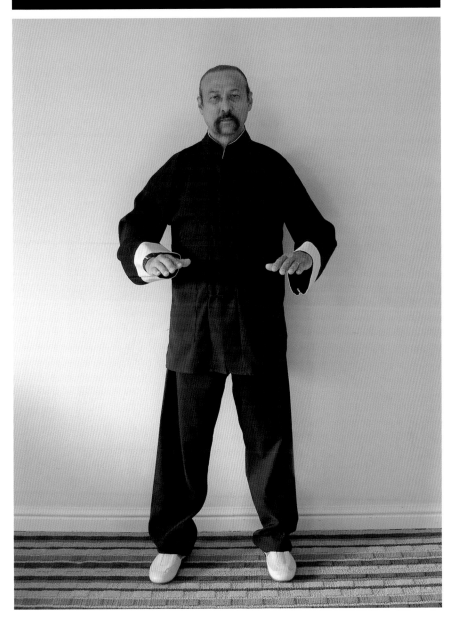

Inhaling slowly lower arms to sternum.

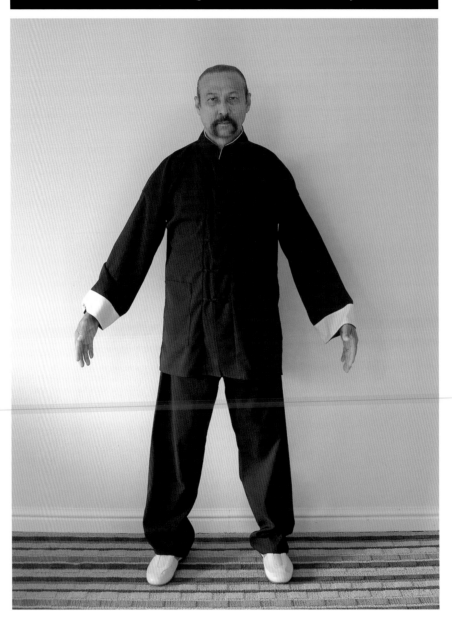

Exhale slowly rotate palms to face upward, continue exhaling lowering arms.

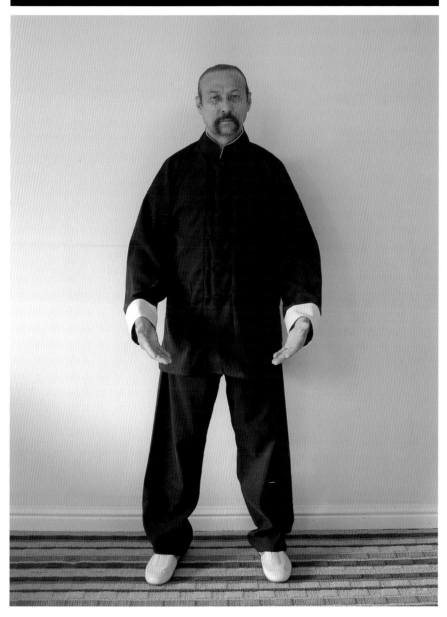

Inhaling slowly, lower both arms to position shown.

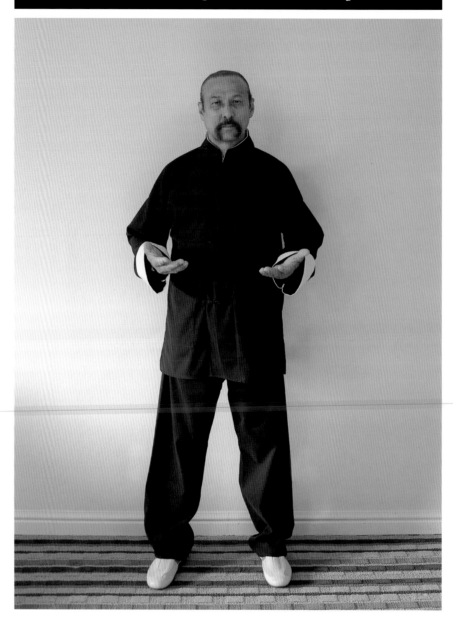

Inhaling slowly as you continue to raise both arms so that both palms are facing upward.

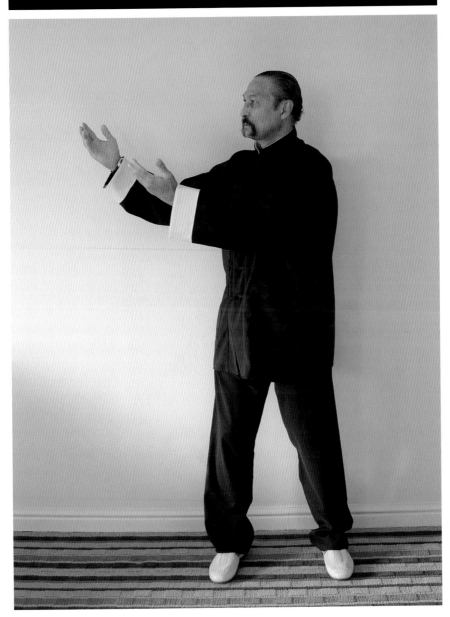

Exhaling slowly while moving arms.

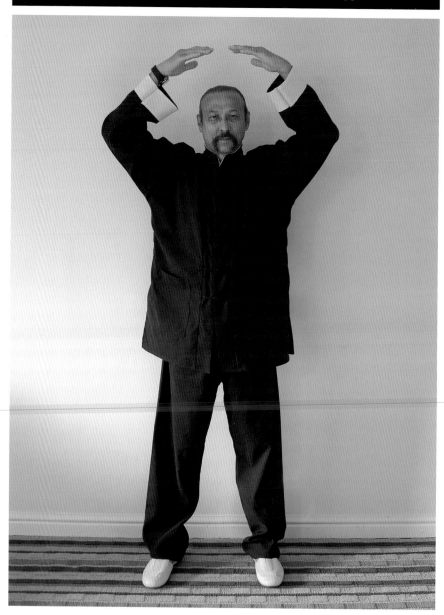

Inhale as both arms are raised until directly overhead.

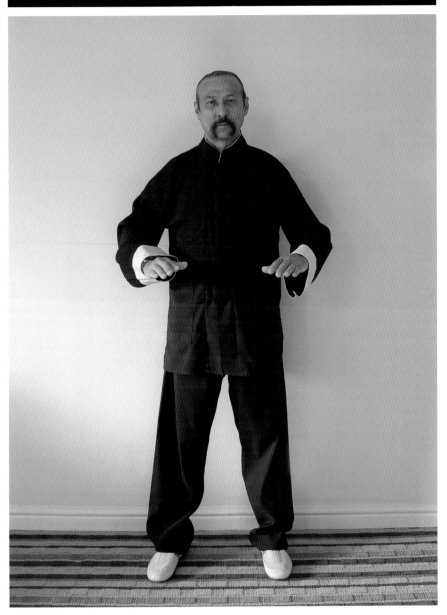

Continue inhaling slowly while lowering both arms.

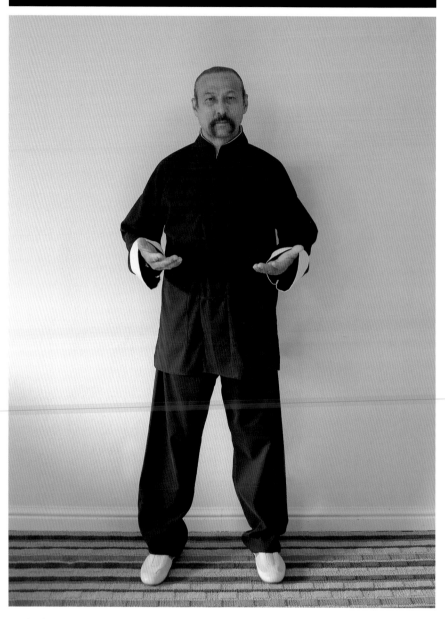

Exhale as both palms are rotated and raised until facing upward.

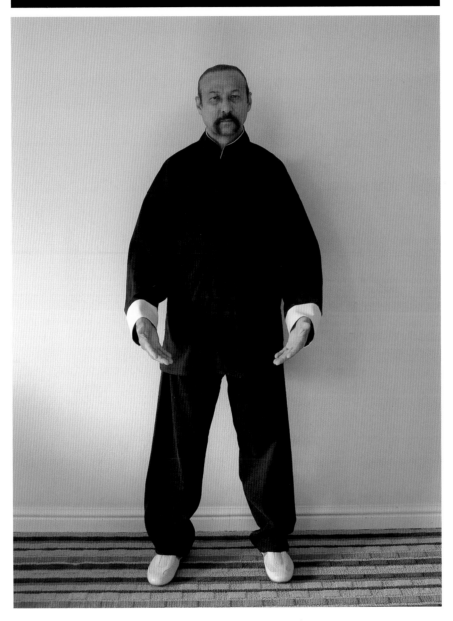

Inhaling slowly lower both arms to position shown.

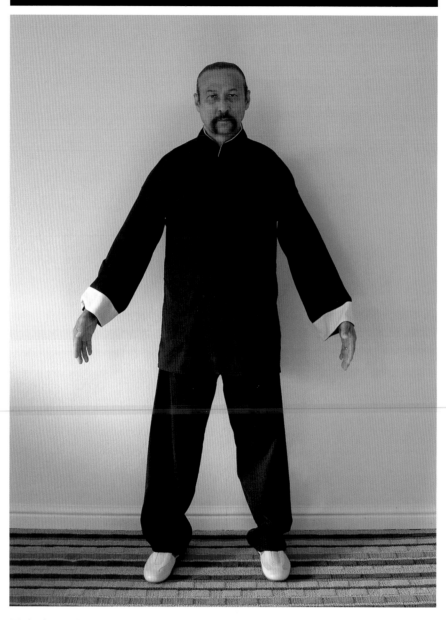

Exhaling slowly move both arms to your sides

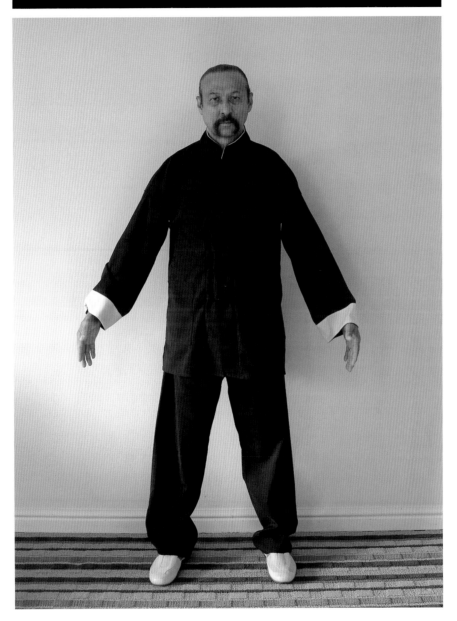

Do not move. Take 9 slow deep breaths.

(END)

Water and Qi

THE HUMAN BODY is made up of a large percentage of water—between eighty and eighty-four percent depending on the person's fluid intake and physical size. Therefore, it is advisable to learn something about the philosophy of Qi Gong and its understanding of the Water element.

An expanse of water that is still or not flowing will eventually become stagnant. Obviously, no energy can be realized from a source that is inactive, even though originally it may have had the potential to provide power.

I recommend that water should never become stagnant, because water that is not flowing, will soon breed disease. Moreover, stagnation of any sort does not bode well. It is the onset of no creation.

When water is stagnant, there is insufficient oxygen to sustain life. Therefore, complex life forms start to perish. Only basic primitive life forms are able to survive in stagnant water, wherein these least developed life forms may even thrive.

We are the same as the water of which we are composed. When we are in a state of stagnation, we become unconscious hosts to attacks by stress. By now, we know that stress will result in some form of disease.

Most importantly, we cannot survive without clean pure drinking water.

And we need our Qi, our life force, to be moving.

If not, we then become stagnated. Stagnation surely causes spiritual, mental and physical stress. Hence, our spirit, mind, and bodies are at the mercy of disease. Disease does not respect nor care for anyone regardless of social status or standing.

Fast flowing water creates the conditions for potential energy. This potential energy will eventually decrease or dissipate because it

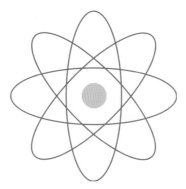

expends itself unless replenished from another source. At some point, the water becomes stagnant and results in a waste of what could have been useful energy. This same condition occurs with Qi in the body.

Water that is directed to move in a disciplined and controlled manner will realize its potential in a harvestable and plentiful state because its energetic source will be governed by the requirements placed upon it. (Think of the water that flows from your faucets when you turn the handle.)

Capacity and capability increase or decrease in a disciplined and controlled system ensuring that water (or whatever the commodity) is accessible. Because we are composed mostly of water, our human systems require a constant replenishment of energy that can be attained by adopting the controlled-moving-water concept—lest we stagnate and invite disease.

From time to time, we demonstrate signs and symptoms of poor health. Often, these are displayed unconsciously, and even if we are aware of them, we sometimes try to hide or disguise such indications from others. These signs are an excellent indicator that something is having a radical effect on our health—often at times, at a level beyond our control.

In due course, the symptoms manifest to such an extent that we are unable to function properly. Thereafter, we portray the distinct signals of an individual under stress.

However, as you now know, there is a very easy-to-achieve preventative measure to deal with this problem. And the value of this measure is that it is ultimately the most effective, least expensive and non-invasive when compared to modern medical and psychiatric remedies. Furthermore, Qi Gong is free of the stressful side effects of these other forms of treatment.

Practicing Qi Gong strengthens our internal coping mechanisms. It also prevents further damage to our health by improving the functions of all our systems:

METABOLIC SYSTEM:

Qi Gong improves one's metabolism, an important function for health, by enabling the activity of tissue cells.

ANABOLIC METABOLISM:

Qi Gong increases one's ability to resist degeneration, and in doing so, prolongs life by decreasing cholesterol levels in blood.

DIGESTIVE SYSTEM:

Qi Gong improves the nervous systems and therefore its functional activity and performance by improving the digestive system.

CIRCULATORY SYSTEM:

Qi Gong regulates blood circulation providing a more effective system, thereby offering a type of preventative action, with regard to constipation.

RESPIRATORY SYSTEM:

The gentle, quiet slowing down of the number of breaths taken while practicing Qi Gong, results in a state of suppressed cerebral cortex activity. This reduced unconscious excitation of the brain's parameters is a required state for self-healing, specifically for pneumonia, bronchitis, asthma and tuberculosis.

Qi Gong Disposition:

By practicing Qi Gong, a condition of calm is derived that provides a good effect on human dispositions. Individuals will be less easily upset by their daily tasks and any other problems. Reducing the development of emotional states such as anger, can prevent some types of heart complaints.

We should try to limit any further development of our stress-related problems. This can be achieved by researching and seeking whatever assistance is available, regardless of the discipline involved, because some aid is better than no help at all.

However, adapting a tried and tested system that is easy to use and dynamic in its results, is preferable. The focused, controlled, quiet breathing, accompanied by synchronized, slow, gentle, stylized movements of LAMAS Qi Gong have been proven to be of great efficacy.

Nutrition and Qi

The universal input and output orifices of the human body present main entry points for disease to freely gain access.

The mouth is the path used in consuming food (input).

The anus is the path utilized in excreting waste products (output).

The genitalia are the path for our reproductive system.

Disease will and may enter any or all of the body's orifices.

The intent of disease is to invade the body. And there are many paths beside these by which it may accomplish this mission. One example is via the body's largest organ, the skin. Disease may enter through any other body apertures and any area that may be damaged or prone to the attack of "Perverse Qi."

If we understand the pervasive, invasive and subtle means by which the body is generally threatened, it is fairly obvious, (although surprising to many), that food can and does cause the onset of stress. Yet sages have known since ancient times how important a role proper food plays in the human health. If we make poor choices in our diet, we may simply provide another avenue for the entry of stress into the body.

What is happening today is that the problem is becoming so pervasive that an increasing awareness is growing in modern society. For example, let us highlight another report taken from a popular media source. A *Daily Mail* article on January 3, 2008, reported that the British government estimated that some 70,000 lives a year could be saved by a healthier diet. Political reporter Daniel Martin wrote, "One in ten premature deaths could be prevented if Britons reduced the amount of salt, sugar and fat they eat." He went on to say that the Cabinet Office suggested people were killing themselves by not eating a more healthy diet that included more fruits, vegetables, fiber and fish oil. The report concluded that people put themselves at greater risk from cancer and heart disease through poor dietary habits. The article continued that scientists estimate one third of cardiovascular cases and a quarter of cancer deaths may be diet-related. It noted that fast food consumption and the use of prepared food are rising at an incredible pace and attributes poor dietary habits to the rise in the rate of diabetes, expected to increase by fifteen percent between 2001 and 2010, with more than half of that due to increasing obesity rates.

I contend that we must take immediate steps to offer resistance to stress by making changes in our lifestyles. Unless we do so, the internal discord that our organs endure because of incorrect eating habits will cause our health to decline in a downward spiral.

Food-generated stress and the path that this vibration takes, have never before been researched, nor chronicled until the publication of this book.

A particular characteristic of thermal stress is its ability to rise upward. This is due to the potential difference of the Yang (Hot) Fire character of stress, which has a rising propensity, and will trigger the increase of internal thermal heat.

This proclivity is completely opposite to the Yin (Cool) nature of Water, which has a predisposition to sink downward and is inherently cool. Thus, it is referred to as Yin. Clean water is therefore very restorative.

From the Qi Gong culture and Oriental viewpoint, stress has a distinct Yang feature. Such a stress characteristic is similar to some types of cultivated Qi, which also have a Yang element.

Yang Qi is said to be rising Qi. It is the opposite of Yin Qi, which is said to be sinking Qi.

Yang Qi is said to rise, spiralling upward in the human body, at the same time and with similar speed to Yin Qi, which sinks and spirals downward in the body.

Foods have both Yang and Yin traits or factors. After various internal processes, including full digestion, the spleen transforms received food. It alters the food completely, so that what had been consumed becomes a component of a particular element of Qi. This Spleen transformed Qi is then transported to the Lungs, to await other internal functions. Simply put, food forms one of the constituents of Qi.

The hygienic preparation of food and the varieties of food eaten, all form a major part of my strategy for retaining good health. After all, food is a means by which our internal systems help to enrich the body's depleted nutritional levels.

Stress attacks caused by poor consumables will in time mutate into physical and/or organ dysfunction.

Below are some foods that aid in the reduction of the initial mental stress hormone attacks:

- All types of oily fish
- Fresh ginger
- Wild rice
- Very low-fat milk
- Oats
- Romaine lettuce
- Pasta
- Avocado pears
- Couscous
- Some herbal teas
- Root of a Siberian plant namely "Rhodiola"
- Edible plants with dark colors and vibrant growth

Harmful microbes thrive in an acidic system and do not flourish in an alkaline system. The more acidic foods and beverages that one consumes, the more hospitable one's system is to disease. Hence, you are advised to eat more alkaline than acidic foods to create an internal environment that is less likely to host diseases.

Alkaline Fruits:
- Apples & Avocados
- Bananas & Berries
- Cantaloupe, Cherries & Currants
- Dates & Figs
- Grapes & Guavas
- Kumquats & Loquats
- Mangos
- Melons
- Olives
- Papayas, Peaches, Pears, Persimmons
- Pomegranates
- Pumpkin
- Raisins
- Radish & Romaine lettuce
- Sauerkraut, Soybeans, Spinach & Sprouts
- Squash & Turnips
- Sweet potatoes
- Tamarind & Tomatoes
- Watercress
- Yams

Alkaline Vegetables:
- Alfalfa Sprouts, Artichokes & Asparagus
- Bamboo Shoots, Beans, Beets & Broccoli
- Cabbages, Carrots, Celery & Cauliflower
- Chard, Chicory & Cucumber
- Dill & Dock
- Eggplant & Endive
- Garlic
- Horseradish
- Jerusalem Artichokes
- Kale
- Leeks & Lettuce

- Mushrooms
- Okra, Onions & Oyster Plant
- Parsley, Parsnips & Peas

Alkaline Dairy:
- Acidophilus Milk, Buttermilk, Yogurt & Whey

Alkaline Grains:
- Quinoa
- Buckwheat & Millet are considered either neutral or alkaline

Alkaline Nuts:
- Almonds, Chestnuts (roasted) & Coconut (fresh)

Alkaline—Other:
- Agar, Honey & Kelp (edible, Teas)

Here is my A to Z list of guidelines to prevent, reduce and finally eliminate many of the problems caused by incorrect eating habits.

a) Avoid all fast foods.
b) Broccoli should be eaten raw or lightly steamed.
c) Carrots should be served always whole, raw and cold.
d) Drink hot liquids. Water purity is essential.
e) Eat lots of fully cooked fresh seafood.
f) Fruit fresh daily is critical to good health.
g) Garlic and onions are good for curing/seasoning.
h) Honey is perfect to enjoy a sweet repast.
i) Indian maize or corn, of good quality, are healthy.
j) Just steam dark green, leafy vegetables.
k) Keep bread whole meal or stone ground.
l) Indulge in cheese once per week.

m) Milk should be kept to a minimum if female and over forty.

n) Never eat everything on your plate.

o) Oily fish boosts brain immunity.

p) Peppers are best fresh.

q) Quinine is useful to reduce muscle cramps.

r) Reduce or forgo using fungi as food.

s) Shallots or spring onions are very good.

t) Tomatoes should be cooked at high temperatures.

u) Unfiltered water is a major factor in disease.

v) Vegetables are best lightly steamed.

w) Walnuts offer protection from cancers.

x) Xtra care chewing your food twenty to thirty times is important.

y) Yes to fish. No to beef.

z) Zest of lemons is ok in drinking water

After eating your food, the digestion process involves the energetic Yin element which will transmigrate the Qi element to the Spleen. After undergoing transformation here, it will be transported to the Lungs. This Yin element is cold in nature, and the Qi is said to be sinking in essence and direction. It is opposite to the Yang element.

However, since we are only concerned here with stress and its various factors, it is unnecessary to follow the Yin element any further. Stress has a Yang feature as its natural characteristic. The path of stress is therefore energetic. Its Qi element, which is said to be rising both in essence and the direction, will take the path of least or easiest resistance.

The Yang stress element path is orbital. It first follows the food we have eaten, then the path of digestion. Consequently, the Yang essence transmigrates in an upward direction.

We can visualize it as a nebulous force carried by the flow of blood. It can be viewed as an energetic element, entering via the vena cava, travelling upward, arriving and entering into the right atrium (a pump in the upper chamber of the heart). This energetic source then passes through the atrioventricular valve to the right ventricle (a lower chamber which is a muscular contraction type pump). Eventually, it joins the oxygen-enriched blood in the left atrium (another pump in one of the chambers of the heart).

Thereafter, a contingency occurs and transmission of thermal heat is generated. The energetic component of the Yang element becomes part of the blood flow.

This unwanted energetic Yang element could be ameliorated by the transmission of heterodynated Qi (hetrodynation is a process where the electron space cloud within the human dipole envelope is overcome by focused thought). This particular objective is obtained only by practicing LAMAS Qi Gong, of which Lion's Tail Qi Gong is an important part.

Here are seven more ways—compatible with conventional, complementary and alternative therapy—to reduce the effects of stress:

1. Multi-nutrient supplements (in very controlled dosage)
2. Natural dietary fiber (as part of your daily intake)
3. Digestive tract manipulation (massage)
4. Antispasmodic colonic treatment (colonic irrigation)
5. Tests for food allergies (checks for intolerance)
6. Spinal manumission (Qi Gong manipulation)
7. A less stressful lifestyle (reduction of stress causing factors)

Activity: Stress-Reducing Nutrition

Keep notes or log and also monitor everything you eat and drink for meals and snacks.

Circle the items that are alkaline. (Generally, fruits and vegetables are alkaline.)

If something that you ate is not listed above, consult a book at a health food store, or search alkaline/acidic food lists online. Each day, estimate what percentage of your intake is alkaline.

If you are typical, your goal should be to increase your intake of alkaline foods. Ideally, eighty percent is advised.

Begin adjusting portions and types of food you eat to increase alkalinity. For example, eat only half a baked potato instead of a whole potato, and increase your portion of green vegetables. Drink green tea instead of coffee and wherever possible, eliminate coffee entirely.

Reduce or eliminate junk foods and for snacks, strive to eat raw carrots and almonds.

Experiment with alkaline foods that are new to you. Never had millet? Try it as part of your breakfast. Then stock up on it and try millet in a new recipe.

Strive to try familiar alkaline foods in creative ways. For example, utilize orange slices instead of croutons on your garden salad. Or, add spinach or sprouts to your scrambled eggs.

Your taste buds will adjust to the change in eating patterns. After several weeks of eating wholesome foods, your cravings for foods with "empty calories" will decrease.

Different people notice varying benefits from decreasing their intake of acidic foods.

Some notice more supple skin, more efficient bowel movements, increased energy, decreased cravings, disappearance of heartburn, and so on.

After you have increased your intake of alkaline foods and beverages, make a list of all the improvements you have noticed.

When you feel tempted to fall back into old, unhealthy eating habits, re-read your list of personal improvements.

You are advised to review your list especially when feeling stressed, for that is when we tend to indulge in less nutritious foods and drinks.

Activity: Stress Reduction Chart

First, create a chart that divides your days into two-hour increments, or whatever blocks of time best represent your usual day.

Several times daily, (once at a minimum), note internal and external causes of stress that occurred in each block of time. (Remember that both pleasant and unpleasant stimuli can cause stress.)

In the Reaction column, document how you responded or behaved.

In the final column, write how you plan to react so that you can reduce the effects of stress under similar circumstances in the future.

On the next page is an excerpt from one person's Stress Reduction Chart.

Please do not forget that you can increase your health and well-being at any time by making better choices. Changing one's lifestyle is worth while as, once again, we find confirmed even in the popular media.

The medical correspondent for the *Daily Telegraph* pointed out in an article on January 8, 2008 that the effects of four common behaviors (smoking, drinking, lack of exercise, and poor diet) are a deadly combination. The article highlighted the work of Professor Kay-Tee-Khaw, a gerontologist at Cambridge University, who found that a healthy lifestyle can increase a person's lifespan by as much as fourteen years. Scientists determined that those who do not smoke, drink moderately, eat healthy foods and keep physically active, can extend the length of their lives by up to seventeen percent. Professor Khaw's study is published in the journal *PloS Medicine*. He and his team surveyed 20,244 men and women living in Norfolk, England in the mid-

Monday	Cause	Reaction	Future Action
1:00-3:00 p.m.	Mom forgot to phone me.	Negative thoughts.	Must phone Mom.
3:00-5:00 p.m.	Didn't finish writing month-end report.	Drank a pot of coffee, stayed late at work.	Will daily do my Qi Gong breathing and Color visualization.
5:00-7:00 p.m.	Too tired to prepare dinner for my family.	Picked up fast food on the way home.	Stock up on Fresh Fruit, easily cooked Vegetables.
7:00-11:00 p.m.	Tired, stressed-out.	Watched TV until bedtime.	Sign up for cooking class, do Lion's Tail, move TV out of the bedroom.

1990s. When in 2006, an average of eleven years later, the researchers re-contacted those who took part, they found that 1,987 had died since they were first interviewed. Those who combined smoking and drinking with failure to exercise, and lack of fruit and vegetables in their diets, were four times more likely to have died than those who had lived healthier lifestyles.

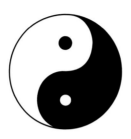

Part Four:

More on Qi Gong

Universal Qi Flow in Buildings

- Do work or leisure time activities make you feel exhausted or overwhelmed?
- Do your work and home life suffer?
- Does juggling several tasks leave you unable to fully accomplish any of them?
- Does it take you more time than it normally would to complete tasks?
- Honestly, do you fear that what you set out to achieve might end up a shambles?

IF YOUR ANSWER to any of these questions is, "Yes," then you are surely suffering from stress.

It may very well be that you are unaware of real, useful, successful techniques to overcome these feelings. On the other hand, perhaps you were lulled into one of the various and possibly well-intended philosophies, that do not offer the effectiveness which one requires for real healing. Some of these may have seemed stimulating at first. Such philosophies or techniques may have even provided you with some temporary satisfaction and amusement, allowing periods of the "feel-good" factor.

However, when reality kicks in, you may realize that the measure or yardstick which you employed, had only provided the opportunity for stress to come to its full health-destructive maturity.

Health is not to be confused with fitness. One can possess a good measurable level of fitness, but may have some yet unexposed, non-symptomatic, hibernating disease, whatever its origin.

Please do not confuse a state of good health with a good level of fitness.

SICK BUILDING SYNDROME (SBS)

The harmony and balance that are offered by the philosophy of Qi Gong are highly desirable to offset Sick Building Syndrome (SBS).

Sick Building Syndrome is a condition of stress induced into the occupants of a man-made structure. It is caused by an energetic imbalance within the edifice in which one resides or is employed.

When a building is out of harmony with the environment, it causes a form of disruption of the universal Qi flow (not to be confused with the Qi flowing within an organic being). Such environmental imbalance creates discord and allows Perverse Qi to develop.

The shape and color of a properly conceived building will merge and blend into the surrounding plant life and contours of the land. Such enlightened design encourages the continuity and permanence of smooth Qi flow. This movement of harmony and balance is similar to the flux that connects the Three Treasures—which govern our ethos, thoughts and actions.

Such harmony resonates in the natural balance between those environmental factors with which we interweave our daily lives. We are part of this living tapestry. And it is all the more invigorating because we have joined in a natural way of living/working without destroying nature's visually rewarding aspects.

How you think, feel, and behave has much to do with Qi flow in the buildings you occupy. Happiness and success can originate from a state of well being both at home and at work. Changing our lifestyles to cultivate environmentally friendly, harmonious energy systems around us will encourage smooth Qi flow at a micro-molecular level. Smooth Qi flow prevents various forms of stress.

You can achieve significant and tangible results using a systematic and daily approach, with Qi Gong practice as the main format. In addition, selecting the best location for any facility in which you spend time, will help to improve your health.

Look at the places where you live, work, or play. Sensing the emanating vibrations will indicate (to anyone versed in the Wind/Water

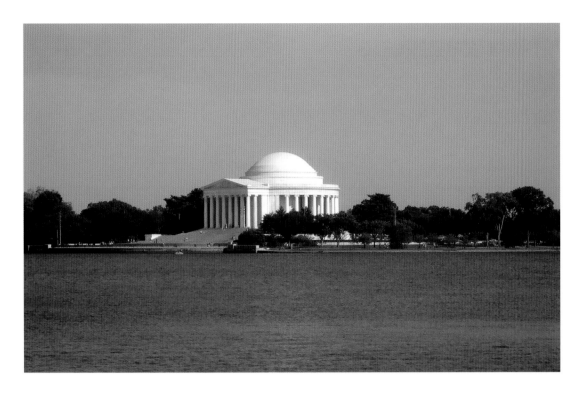

principle) the best location for the bath, shower, toilet, sink, bidet, Jacuzzi, swimming pool, sauna, and so forth.

I cannot emphasize strongly enough that colors, materials and the positions of objects, furniture and other personal belongings, play a vital role in the relief of stress generated by the Sick Building Syndrome.

Using a simplified Ba-Gua template (see following page) you may be able to encourage the flow of smooth Qi through the buildings where you live, work, or play.

Lay the Ba-Gua template on a floor plan or architect's drawings with the blue sector facing true north.

Make adjustments in the layout, wherever possible, to ensure that the rudimentary energy of your personal space is adequate. You can enhance good thoughts, actions and Qi flow by becoming conscious of the ways in which positive energy may be enhanced by proper décor.

For example, the placement of the front door can support or sabotage the intent of the occupants of that building.

For a business premises, the main entrance positioned…

- To the left, signifies aspects of knowledge. This entrance is called Ken.
- In the center, promotes business and/or career prospects. This entrance is called K'an.
- To the right, depicts directed energy of helpful persons. This entrance is called Chyan.

These locations—left, center, and right—define three of the corners of the Ba-Gua.

For a home, the main entrance positioned…

- To the left side, represents wealth.
- In the center, promotes career and professional aspiration.
- To the right, signifies marriage, a settled home life, and good relationships.

Whatever use of the building, the front door and foyer or hallway should be welcoming, well lit and spacious. The door should open inwards.

The placement and type of furniture and décor in the interior space can also either hinder or promote Qi flow. To promote smooth Qi flow in any building …

- Avoid placing furniture where it protrudes into pathways and corridors.
- Use mirrors to add continuity and the flow of good Qi.
- Keep the home and office light and bright.
- Hang chimes to create sound and movement and crystals to refract light—creating a calm state.
- Have healthy plants to increase general harmony and provide a visually restful environment. Plants should not be

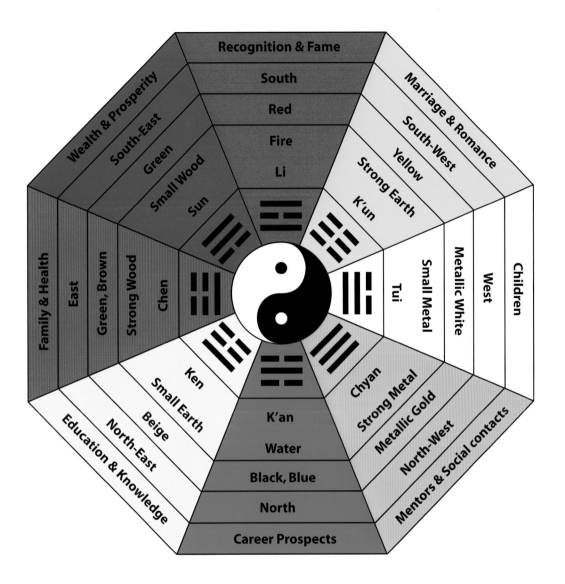

sharp or pointed. Spikey plants represent an inducement to arguments and disagreements. Cacti, yucca, spider plants, and mother-in-law's tongue are not recommended. Chinese lantern, Philodendron, Goosefoot, Birds' Nest Fern, Fuchsia, Hibiscus, Bougainvilleas and African Violets are desirable because they have rounded leaves. If your plants are in the corners of a room, keep them softly illuminated.

- Make sure that furniture or other features in the room do not cause you headaches or backaches.

- Wherever possible, avoid fittings and decor with sharp edges.
- Beds should not be placed directly under large beams or rafters, or in front of, or facing doors either vertically or horizontally.
- Always keep the head of the bed clear of cupboards, shelves, ornaments, etc.
- Ensure that there are no electrical cables or connections around or near the head of the bed.
- Avoid mirrors directly facing the bed, that is, at the foot or head of the bed.
- Round and oval mirrors are best for Qi flow.
- The correct location of mirrors can prevent energy losses. Well placed mirrors recycle good energy that enters through open windows and puts it to good use. Mirrors can also enhance the positive existing energetic attributes within the building, and that which issues from the occupants.
- Mirrors should be clear and untarnished.
- Use as large a mirror as possible for the space you have.
- Hang mirrors at the ends of corridors.
- Windows should be open at some time each day and kept clean.
- Give the building a name, which suits your personality.
- Use fragrances to add to the general feeling of well being.
- Keep toilet seats closed when not in use.
- Ornaments, accessories, furniture, fabrics, etc. should be well crafted from natural materials.
- Outside, wind chimes provide a peaceful vibration.
- Keep the immediate landscape as natural as possible.
- Position the building's water features and ornaments as per the instructions of a Qi Gong exponent who has old knowledge of the Tao Tang concept of the art of Feng Shui.

Eight easy ways toward a happier home life are the following:

1. Avoid clutter.
2. Neatly store anything not in regular or weekly use.
3. Sell, give away, donate, or discard all possessions that are not of any use.
4. Eliminate collections of papers and magazines.
5. Clean and organize drawers, closets, cupboards, and wardrobes.
6. Employ colors that enhance your personal energy levels.
7. Clean and rearrange your refrigerator on a weekly basis.
8. Mirrors, plants, furniture, and colors can add or reduce the cosmic energy levels that are part of the process of success.

When asked to improve smooth Qi flow in a home or workplace, I use an original family Ba Gua divination board.

However, you do not have to use a Ba Gua board. Just follow what your senses are attracted to. This will be your basic guide to using colors in the décor, furnishings and clothing that reflect the energy you wish to convey and, most importantly, which you desire or need to absorb. (A color might appear to you during meditation. Use it in the décor and settings of your environment.)

The colors below represent the ascending value of the colors that one visualizes during static Qi Gong meditation. (Static Qi Gong is done without external body movement)

- Black: Distortion of reality—Inner fear—Limitations
- Brown: Grounding—Stability—Challenges
- Pink: Inner strength—Inner power
- Red: Yang energy denoting Outer strength—Power—Passion
- Orange: Mental discipline—Expansive—Cheerful
- Yellow: Mental clarity—Wisdom—Organizational skills

- Cyan: Emotional Clarity — Adjustment
- Green: Balance — Peace — Serenity — Adaptability
- Dark Blue: Relaxing — Establishes parameters — Responsibility
- Light Blue: Honesty — Sincerity — Perfectionist — Trust — Sensitivity
- Indigo: Cleansing — Inner vision — Meditation — Composure
- Magenta: Warmth — Passion — Communication — Emotion
- Violet: Inspirational — Positive Innovative — Grace
- White: Purity — Higher purpose — Objectivity
- Gold: Divine inspiration — Spiritual evolution — Vibrant spirituality

To summarize, you can conquer stress on two fronts: breath and lifestyle.

Learn to use your breath correctly by practicing a daily modality that's been used for thousands of years.

This ancient, wholesome and dynamic technique does not require drugs, a particular religious doctrine or any form of political dogma.

Qi Gong in my opinion is the best practice. Moreover, Lion's Tail Qi Gong can increase and enhance internal Light.

Secondly, you are advised to change your lifestyle if it is causing stress factors that are damaging your health and therefore your life.

It is up to you to alter whatever is damaging your health, even if it entails a reduction or abstinence of your worldly desires including: changing your employment, adjusting your choice and volume of food consumed and beverage intake.

Also, take the necessary steps now to remove any unwanted energies or undesirable energetic propensities from your home and/or place of employment.

Qi: Source of Internal Light

So, you have been practicing Lion's Tail on a daily basis and have enjoyed the slow, gentle, deep breathing technique for at least fifteen minutes. Did you know that you have been cultivating Qi?

Qi Gong, literally translated, means "skill of breath." Breath control combined with soft gentle movements will provide an individual with the mechanism to release physical tension and eliminate the physical stress response. This stress response, if left unattended, will eventually lead to some form of health complaint. Further, it will lead to symptoms and signs that are at most times completely unconnected with the initial sensation.

Qi Gong breathing—together with dynamic visualization and color guided meditation techniques—when practiced on a daily basis, cultivate Universal Qi. Many Qi Gong practitioners of different and varied Qi Gong traditions often mistakenly refer to Cultivated Qi as the life-force. Only True Qi and/or Prenatal Qi have the ability to increase Longevity.

True Qi, or the life force, of the practitioner is a bio-chemically produced microcosmic, electromagnetic field which is changed into an intrinsic highly energized source of internal Light. (Just a few years ago, researchers discovered that the large intestine or colon produces a form of light. For ages, Chinese culture has said that all organs produce different hues of internal light.)

It is a worldwide and universally accepted idea that according to Chinese culture we have five paired organs. It is my personal opinion that we have six paired organs. (Now I've put the cat out among the pigeons!)

These are the six paired organs:

1) Heart + Small Intestine
2) Lung + Large Intestine
3) Kidney + Urinary Bladder
4) Spleen + Stomach
5) Liver + Gall Bladder
6) Pericardium + Triple Heater/Burner/Warmer. Only one of these produces light. The Pericardium emits a silvery colored light.

The Light in our bodies comes from a source. I suggest that this internal Light is created from within all our organs.

Each Yin organ is paired with a Yang organ. Yin and Yang energies are always in opposition. Within this duality lies sickness and health.

Depending on an individual's lifestyle, the energetic element produced by the passage of Qi emits internal Light from each of the paired Organs. A true medical Intuitive should be able to "see" via this internal light, any previously undetected indication of some of the multitude of effects of stress-causing "Perverse Qi."

This emitted Light is the internal healing life force that resides within each of the paired organs.

Stress decays the internal Light and weakens the human constitution. This weakened condition causes disease. The decrease in energy levels also creates an executive interrupt, triggering the release of cerebral emitted neuron instructions. After an undefined period, the outcome of such confused signals may produce a dysfunctional or depressed individual.

Stress is a no-Light condition. In contrast, people in a state of no-stress would be in a state of enhanced Light.

To achieve or increase internal Light requires the implementation of Qi Gong meditation and visualization. Preliminary information and guidance for the initial practices and principles of LAMAS Qi Gong are provided within these pages. More in-depth and highly

The frequency of internal "Light" is not similar in MHz., nor in sign or signature, to the frequency of additive colors generated by the internal Organs of humans.

WOOD Liver Yin Organ Zang Function	Green Awakening— Awareness Calming	Color of "Light" Cyan— Gall Bladder Yang Organ Fu function
SUN—FIRE Heart Yin Organ Zang Function	Red Uplifting— Freedom—Liberty Internal Energy	Color of "Light" Crimson— Small Intestine Yang Organ Fu Function
EARTH Spleen Yin Organ Zang Function	Brown Reassurance— Harmony—Balance	Color of "Light" Grey— Stomach Yang Organ Fu Function
WATER Kidneys Yin Organ Zang Function	Blue Energetically Deficient Change of Diet	Color of "Light" Cerulean— Urinary Bladder Yang Organ Fu Function
METAL—GOLD Lungs Yin Organ Zang Function	White Stimulation— Interest—Direction Enlightenment	Color of "Light" White— Large Intestine Yang Organ Fu Function
AIR Triple Warmer	Colorless Heat/Energy Stress Elimination	Color of "Light" Silver— Pericardium Zang Fu Functions

informative data (not associated with stress) may further be obtained via LAMAS Qi Gong seminars, workshops and group classes.

I believe if someone were in a state of no-stress, his or her organs would be in a state of reasonably good health. Therefore, by cultivating additional Qi reserves, people have an opportunity and ability to enjoy better health.

Our internal Light is representative of the strength of our life force. Thus, to encourage and enhance this source of Light, I suggest practicing (ShiQi) Lion's Tail Qi Gong.

Travelling along a path of enlightenment brings one closer to the source. Being closer to the source is simple, but is not easy for some people, as it entails living a life that is truly balanced.

A balanced lifestyle requires patience, calm, and forethought. To gain spiritual, mental and physical equilibrium is to live by the basic decent principles that are applicable to any human being:

- Do good deeds regardless of the outcome.
- Do good works without hoping to gain political or religious recognition and acclaim.
- Think good thoughts. They are the building blocks of spiritual and heavenly evolution.

Unhealthy deeds, works and thoughts keep you in bondage. Such unhealthy components are developed and maintained in denial.

Negative deeds, works, and thoughts create a state of un-ease.

A state of un-ease is a state of dis-ease.

Avoid deeds, works and thoughts that cause distress.

Removing yourself from distressing environments is a vital step to reclaiming inner control.

Make this separation at both the mental and physical levels.

To retract physically is to first retract mentally.

Mental retraction allows the development of a stable internal environment.

Wherever possible create a positive, meditative and stable environment.

The alternative to employing effective methods of stress elimination, is a lifestyle of pain, along with various mental and physical complaints, constant internal health problems, unnecessary visible aging, the loss of vitality and unexplained, anti-social behavior, along with a host of other issues.

If you do nothing else, learn and practice proper breathing and you will quickly begin noticing a reduction in your body's stress levels.

Relax and stay calm.

Relax and seek serenity.

Relax. Life doesn't have to be stressful.

Before we are born, that is just prior to birth and during the first few seconds that we enter this world, we are unaware and unconscious of how we breathe.

We use a primal form of abdominal breathing—the same form you used when you were in your mother's body.

But a few seconds after birth, our lungs quickly take over breathing, replacing what was a natural prenatal function.

The connection or similarity between prenatal breathing and Qi Gong breathing is simply this. By breathing deeply, we highly oxygenate our blood supply to a far higher degree than what is the norm. In so doing, we encourage a smoother flow of Qi, since blood attracts and carries Qi during its cycle.

Bio-energy is the byproduct of smooth Qi flow. Physical external movement is not necessary to cultivate Qi. All movement is externally quiescent. However, during Qi Gong breathing practice, a process quietly massages the viscera of the organs inside the body. By breathing gently and slowly, and quietly guiding our breath into the Lower Dantien, we gradually cultivate Universal Qi. (The Lower Dantien is an area in the front of the body about three cun's width below the navel. One cun is equivalent to the length of a single knuckle on a finger.)

Cultivated Qi produces an internal biochemical effect, which in turn creates a type of bio-energy. This bio-energy is a by-product of the controlled focus that is employed in the Qi Gong practice, in order to encourage a uni-directional movement of the cultivated Qi.

Cultivated Qi tends to flow simultaneously in every direction, in and out of our entire being. This flow is due to the internal flux changes.

However, the advantage of practicing microcosmic Qi Gong breathing technique will, with practice, direct the cultivated Qi to the location where it is required for health rectification.

By diligent practice, along with focused thought and slow, quiet breathing, this bio-energy can eventually be directed (after gaining experience and skills through the practice of LAMAS Qi Gong) to the center of one or both palms (Laogong Qi cavities).

Throughout the process, with both eyes closed, one should visualize the cultivated Qi. You should mentally create a small circle of light. It is either white, or in the case of experienced practitioners, the circle may appear as gold in color.

Just off-center in the middle of each palm, this circle of light will eventually be sensed as a pressing sensation, a dull throbbing, a type of fullness, as a vague itching, or as a very subtle type of aching sensation.

Qi Gong seeks movement within quiescence, and quiescence within movement.

Qi Gong works on The Three Treasures. Internal bio-energy is induced by quiet, soft and continuous deep breathing. Wherever necessary, this balances and depletes, Yang, the Fire (Hot) energy by regenerating the restorative Yin, and the Water energy, derived from hormones and neuro-chemicals.

Bio-energy, called Jeng-Qi (true energy) in Chinese, is the basis for health and longevity.

Taoist science accumulated substantial evidence linking the powers of body and mind, neurology and immunology, using techniques developed to activate that link.

The origin of these specific techniques was Qi Gong, sometimes referred to as "Daoyin."

To achieve balance between Nei-dan (Internal bio-energy) and the Wai-dan (External bio-magnetic fields), two distinct states of self-calm and self-awareness must be attained. These two states formulate the Mind and Body connection and when they are in harmony, true balance will be attained.

During your Qi Gong meditation the linking of Mind and Body may be viewed as becoming one within yourself. When you reach this stage, you will no longer feel this inner separation. Thus, you should have no sensation of reality. Yet you may thereby experience what others have sought without any real success for millennia.

This sense of Oneness is that which you must seek to establish within yourself.

During the experience of Oneness, the high-frequency activity of the cerebral cortex is decreased. This permits the restorative Yin (Water energy) low-frequency oscillation of the parasympathetic nervous system to take control of the body's organs and their functions.

This calm awareness within the self, harmonizes with the low frequency, electromagnetic Earth pulses that boost living biological systems.

Qi Gong Boosts Immunity

OUR IMMUNE SYSTEMS are always at war with germs and microorganisms that constantly invade and attack our bodies.

Humans have two types of immunity: passive and acquired.

Passive immunity is gained from mother's milk. This is automatically primed to offer some resistance to disease, while the infant develops the more powerful system of acquired immunity.

From birth through the first four to five years, our passive immune systems, though not yet fully evolved nor developed, will nonetheless begin to offer rudimentary opposition against disease and try to protect our health. In the very young, it is a matter of fighting for survival. However our passive immune system is a rather fragile and vulnerable means of opposition to disease.

Acquired immunity develops as a response to first time contact with new microorganisms. Its memory is sufficiently capable of recalling past attackers (pathogens) to our bodies, thus creating a bio-chemical defense process against future attacks.

This form of auto-vaccination can only defend against one strain of germ each time. It must first learn, then memorize and then defend against each attack, even by a pathogen producing some characteristics similar to previously encountered pathogens. In the auto-vaccination procedure, our body recognizes invasive elements or substances (antigens), and creates defenses against them.

Our immune system acts like an organic army, capable of sending bio-chemical messages to communicate orders of defense deployment and to engage invasive microorganisms or germs. Hence, it is obvious that our defense system must create a host of bio-defense programs to combat the constant onslaught of countless diseases.

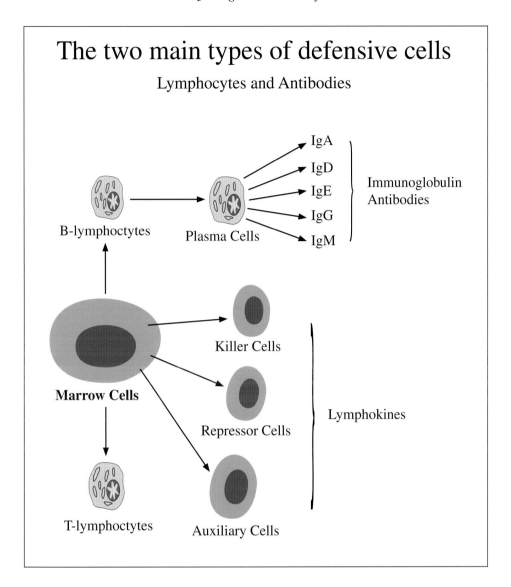

The two main types of defensive cells

Lymphocytes and Antibodies

The lymphatic system is comprised mainly of the spleen, thymus gland, tonsils, bone marrow and other organs. These work in conjunction with the capillaries and lymphatic ducts and glands to drain the clear bodily fluid known as lymph from the body tissue. Lymph then passes into the blood stream.

We have two main types of defensive cells: lymphocytes and antibodies.

Lymphocytes are white blood cells. These originate in the bone marrow.

Antibodies are complex blood protein molecules. They have a branching structure with special surfaces shaped to interlock with invading germs, or the toxins the germs produce, and thereafter neutralize them.

The defensive process does not end there.

Scavenger cells, called macrophages, are continually engaged in a search for any antibody-coated antigens. These macrophages are large cells found in the blood, the lymph, and connective tissues. They remove waste products, harmful microorganisms, and foreign materials.

The production of antibodies depends on two types of lymphocytes.

B-lymphocytes (B-cells) are the first to recognize antigens in the body and the first to produce the antibody reaction. If the same microorganism attacks again, then specific B-cells, specialized for that particular antigen, come into maturation rapidly. These immediately produce large amounts of the appropriate antibodies. But B-cells cannot defend us on their own. They depend on T-lymphocytes.

T-lymphocytes (T-cells) play a significant and direct role in destroying invading organisms. T-cells even attack the body's own cells if they have become infected. T-cells are named after the thymus gland (in the upper chest) from which they evolve, develop, and in which they mature. There are several types of T-cells.

One type of T-cell is the Cytotoxic cell, so-called because of its cell-poisoning ability. Cytotoxic T-cells lock onto particular antigens on the surface of infected cells in much the same way as B-cells do. Cytotoxic T-cells destroy the infected cells by breaking down the outer walls of the pathogen.

There are other T-cells known as "natural killers" that don't need to be programmed. They easily recognize and destroy any foreign materials, whether they've been encountered before or not. Unfortunately, not all cancerous parasites get destroyed.

Helper T-cells are said to switch on B-cells. Suppressor T-cells do the opposite. They switch off B-cells.

The balance between helper T-cells and suppressor T-cells is vital for controlling immunity. Viruses attack the immune system at this point, infecting and destroying helper T-cells.

The Fitness News section in the April 29, 2008 issue of the *Daily Mail* recognized the direct impact of Qi Gong in enhancing our immune systems. It reported that the *British Journal of Sports Medicine* had published a study in which Tai Chi—the traditional Chinese system which was derived from Qi Gong—was found to help people suffering from type-two diabetes. Taiwanese researchers assessed the effects of Tai Chi on the immune system of those who participated in a twelve week study. They found that those patients who engaged in intense physical exercise actually depressed their immune systems, while those who practiced the more moderate Tai Chi strengthened themselves. Glucose levels dropped, while chemicals that boost the immune system doubled, particularly helper T-cells. The article mentioned that a separate study, conducted in Australia, found similar health benefits from Tai Chi and Qi Gong in those who suffer from either diabetes or heart disease.

The expert Qi Gong practitioner employs three vital energy systems or forces to assist in the prevention and reduction of stress-induced ailments and diseases:

1) Respiratory force.
2) Vibration force—oscillations or vibrations for the transfer of Intentional Qi.
3) Mental force—telepathic or mentally transposed energetic processes.

With daily practice of Lion's Tail Qi Gong, anyone can employ Intentional Qi on a self-help basis.

A person need not become very skilled at Qi cultivation to use the commonly employed self-healing "Universal Qi," (not to be confused with "Intentional Qi"). Universal Qi is obtained from Qi Gong practice. It helps the individual in his or her quest for self-help with personal health issues.

On the other hand, it takes many years of dedicated daily practice before a person can develop the means to transmit Intentional Qi in order to assist in the healing process of others.

Final Thoughts and First Steps

It is important to realize that time lost through delaying the use of correct health therapy is a form of cellular procrastination. If you've read this far in this book, but haven't already begun daily practice of Lion's Tail Qi Gong, or haven't made any other positive lifestyle changes, then you are procrastinating. This period of cellular procrastination allows the development of Perverse Qi, an invasive pestilence of stress in whatever forms it takes.

Stress is stealthy and unassuming. It prevents the retaliatory defense mechanisms of our internal systems to offer any worthwhile resistance—especially during the first attack with the release of stress hormones. This period of no-reaction against the attacks of stress permits the stress factors to quicken and thereafter multiply at a molecular level, increasing their exceedingly harmful potential.

The age-old saying that "prevention is better than a cure" is important to recall when under a macro-instruction attack at a bio-chemical level. The prime factor to observe when attempting to remonstrate with stress is first, to accurately detect it. Thereafter, making use of helpful information gained in identifying the true origins of stress. Next, moving to control and suppress its acceleration, thereby presenting opposition to reduce its effects.

In other words, first make an accurate assumption based on a true detection of the complaint. This is accomplished by identifying the real and original cause of the particular stress condition. This analysis will be complementary to whatever healing modality is to be employed.

The healing method may be conventional, complementary, alternative, or any other form of help. However, when this entire process is properly implemented, it will lead you to creating the best possible conditions for a quick and full recovery wherever possible.

In this way, the opportunity to protect your health remains entirely within your own hands.

The stylized form of Qi cultivation presented in this book, comprising meditation and movement, is your best method of self-empowerment for the control, reduction and elimination of stress.

Practicing Lion's Tail (ShiQi) Qi Gong is the Way to secure a longer, healthier and happier life.

There is another age-old saying: "The first step is the hardest to take." Actually, it's not the first step that we dread. It's the infinite number of steps that follow the first step that intimidate us. We fear the unknown. We doubt our abilities to keep on moving forward. If you feel that way, take the first step anyway. You've done so before in other endeavors. So don't delay, and start enjoying the daily practice of Lion's Tail Qi Gong today!

Know that you are taking the first step of a magnificent journey to improved health and well being. You have absolutely nothing to lose. It's joyful to have nothing to lose. Therefore, any gains received are exceptional and most enjoyable.

I've been fully convinced for over a half a century of my life that the daily practice of Qi Gong is the way to a life of achievable good health objectives.

I also sincerely believe that it is in other people's personal interest to have their unique experiences in the pluralistic philosophy and beneficial practice of LAMAS Qi Gong. I believe that all who practice this system will obtain its benefits and values.

My life's passion and spiritual mission is to disseminate this and any such information as widely as possible, so that others will have the opportunity to care for themselves. My goal is to educate and help as many people as possible to become aware of the multitudinous benefits of participating in the daily practice of LAMAS Qi Gong.

If nothing is certain then nothing is impossible. Decisions are only rational if moral, and made with a clear conscience.

Time and time again—being attentive to the fact that stress respects no one and disease can overcome anyone, I understand it is my duty to offer assistance wherever required, helping those who are physically or spiritually compromised.

I have been able to remain focused on the important issues, those that need priority. I do not allow spurious, sporadic thoughts, or random vibrations to trigger an attack of stress.

Human history tells us that we've always had an overriding inclination to close our eyes and accept comforting untruths, rather than open our eyes to disquietude. However, it is only by honestly and courageously facing reality that we allow ourselves the opportunity to really understand a given situation.

No amount of education or learning can shift what we think we "know." However, it also used to be human nature to "know," for example, that the earth was flat.

I will continue to practice. And it is my earnest hope that others would do likewise, allowing no room in ourselves for the damages of stress to develop.

We are all powerless against fate. Apparently, our future has already betrayed us. But our thoughts and emotions are validated by action that brings results. The power of thought flows not in the direction of greatest need, but in the meridian of least resistance.

I shall also continue to do my best practice. And, by maintaining my health, am committed to making myself available to be of meaningful service to others—whenever, wherever, and in whatever way I can.

Qi Gong over Millennia

QI GONG WAS ONCE AN ESOTERIC ART, created and developed over millennia by the sages of times past. They perfected their knowledge and methods as a result of long periods of intensive study, combined with very careful observations of the seemingly random cycles of nature.

46TH CENTURY B.C.

A legendary philosopher king creates the eight Trigrams of the "I Ching" (The Chinese Book of Divination).

A healer in the king's court encourages the king to order sick people to practice a "Great Dance of Life" to improve their health and be cured of diseases. The dance is composed of slow, gradual movements combined with controlled breathing, the true origins of Qi Gong.

The flood of the river Wu sweeps through the area, causing fatalities and a rampant epidemic. Residents included members of the Taotang and LoLo tribes, my ancient ancestors.

CIRCA 1000 B.C.

The term Daoyin is used to refer to the Great Dance of Life.

CIRCA 1020–221 B.C.

Guo Moruo, a well-known historian and president of the Chinese Academy of Sciences, acknowledges authentic records of Qi Gong movements in Chou Dynasty writings.

CIRCA 770 B.C.

A method of moving meditation (controlled breathing combined with stylized physical movement and visualization), or Daoyin exercise, evolves as a means of curing diseases and improving health.

CIRCA 604 B.C.

Lao Tzu is born and later writes the ancient Chinese classic "The Tao Te Ching" (The Classic Way of the Virtue), containing ideas and principles from which TiJi (Tai Chi) will later be derived.

202 B.C.–25 A.D. (WESTERN HAN DYNASTY)

The Daoyin Silk Scroll is illustrated with over forty human figures in different postures, outlined in black and white and painted in color. The figures represent Qi Gong movements.

2ND CENTURY A.D.

Hua Tuo bases his Wuqinxi exercises on Daoyin principles and instructions.

581–906 A.D. (SUI AND THANG DYNASTIES)

Some Daoyin knowledge, movements, and practices evolve into the discipline known as Taijiquan (TiJi or Tai Chi).

20TH CENTURY A.D.

Two world wars, followed by more affordable and convenient modes of transportation expose other cultures to Asian arts and philosophies, including Qi Gong. Clinical studies by Western researchers indicate the health benefits of Qi Gong.

21ST CENTURY A.D.

Presently, Qi Gong classes and derivatives are offered in gyms, health centers and other venues worldwide.

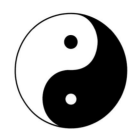

Appendices

Who is LAMAS Qi Gong Grandmaster Lowe?

Born according to the (Lunar calendar 1942), Gregorian calendar 1943, and married in 1966, Grandmaster Lowe is the father of three and grandfather of three. He and his family reside in England, although he travels worldwide to teach Qi Gong, where he offers to help others find the road to recovery of good health.

An Empath, medical intuitive and spiritual Qi healer, Grandmaster Lowe is the lineage holder of LAMAS Qi Gong, earning him the distinction of being the leading authority in this field of Qi Gong.

Grandmaster Lowe is a descendant of the Taotang and LoLo tribes of Ancient China. He has practiced LAMAS Qi Gong, a 3,000-year old and previously esoteric ancestral family art, since he was seven.

Grandmaster Lowe was the only non-American invited to be a presenter and panelist in The First White House Commission on Complementary and Alternative Medical Policy in San Francisco, September 8th, 2000. In February 2002, after his record-breaking, standing-room-only lecture at the University of Colorado, the University Director said of Grandmaster Lowe's presentation, "This was the largest and most popular attended seminar by anyone in the history of the University."

Grandmaster Lowe has been referred to as, "one of the most powerful Qi Gong Masters in the World." He has appeared on various televisions and radio programs and has had articles published in magazines, newspapers, periodicals and journals.

He wrote *The Art of Daoyin* and has produced and been featured in ten instructional Qi Gong DVD's.

Life is Like a Penjing Container

A Traditional LoLo Family Legend
by Lineage holder Grandmaster Lowe

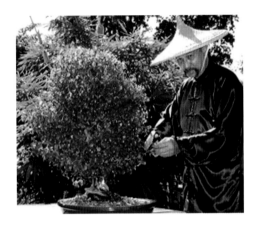

PENJING IS THE ANCIENT Chinese art of landscape miniaturization, and the precursor of the Japanese art of Bonsai. This old LoLo family story was handed down orally around camp fires throughout the ages, and thereafter to me when I was a boy.

An old LAMAS Qi Gong Master knelt in the center of a place of learning within an Emperor's court. He was being observed by many court attendants. However, he was silent, neither speaking nor moving for some protracted minutes even though he could hear the rustle of garments. He also heard the whispers regarding his attitude in the presence of such august persons, and other such comments that were made loud enough to be heard.

He gently picked up an empty almost transparent Penjing container, and slowly began to place in it the stones that he had gathered from the river banks nearby. When the container appeared to be overflowing with the clean smooth stones, he lifted it and looking around the vast meeting place within the Emperor's court, he asked, "Is this container full?"

The court officials and attendees all murmured that obviously the container was full, even a fool could see that. The Master then opened a small sack he had strapped to his waist from which he very carefully removed numerous live seeds he had collected from poppy plants that grew outside the Emperor's palace.

He put the seeds in the Penjing and rattled the transparent container vigorously so the tiny seeds settled in the spaces between the stones. Then, he added more and repeated this procedure until the container appeared quite over-flowing.

The Master again asked the court officials, "Is this container full?" The court officials, monks and their acolytes murmured in complete agreement. Yes, this time the container was definitely full.

The Master next emptied his sack onto the marble floor and a heap of clean very fine sand gushed out. He explained that whilst collecting stones from the river banks, he had painstakingly collected and poured a couple of handfuls of fine, clean sand into his sack. The Master poured some sand into the transparent Penjing container. The sand appeared to trickle into every single tiny area between the stones and poppy seeds, filling the Penjing container to the brim. The old master shook the container, adding sand all the while.

Then, looking around at the gathered frowning audience, he inquired once more, "Is this container full?" The unanimous hearty response was a vibrant, "Yes, Master, the container is completely full now." They said this with great conviction, nodding to each other in the way of the wise. The Master then asked for a bowl of water. He began to slowly pour the water into the transparent Penjing container, just until the water started to overflow and splash onto the marble floor of the meeting place within the Emperor's court.

There were gasps of amazement and a general nodding of heads, a few expelled breaths could be heard and a general buzz echoed throughout.

"This container," said the Master, "is like your life."

"The stones are similar to your achievements and position in life—your family, your dreams, your friends and enemies alike, all your hopes and desires, your innermost secrets, and all those things you would rather not have witnessed by Heaven's light, just heavy stones that will slow your progress to the divine Light.

"The living poppy seeds are your neglected opportunities, your spoken words that hurt others, your childhood days that will never return, physical harm you have inflicted upon others, your time misspent, and all other wrongdoings that will come to haunt you as you get older and sicken. When the fruit of your health will be rotten and decayed, you will not have the health and vigor of the Qi. When the seeds of long life were not put into use, like your treasures locked away in dark places, they see not the light of life.

"The sand represents your Spiritual losses, accumulated when every opportunity that presented itself for you to make proper atonement for your blessings and heavenly gifts was missed. You gathered more of your wrongdoings instead, holding them close to your heart. All the while neglecting to make atonement, and spread the many gifts that were yours, to aid and assist those that were not of your village, not of your kind, and not of your beliefs.

"The water is your time, the balance of what is left of your life and it is running out very quickly.

"Once it overflows not even I can help you, since there appears to be no room for you to take anything else into yourself, perhaps you will become aware of this example.

"However, since you have all agreed that there is no more room within the Penjing container, I will show you what is left for you to save yourself."

The Master lifted up the container and gently blew his soft breath upon the water that had settled upon the top of the contents of the Penjing vessel, saying, "There is still some space within, that which you cannot see. But the breath of life fills the little that is, so like the container, maybe there is still some space within you, such a place for you to make the necessary changes before it's too late."

He lifted the container up higher, so that the sunlight shining through the windows filtered into and apparently filled the transparent container. He looked at the now very still people and said, "The light of life must be allowed to shine within yourselves. Practice the Qi until the Spiritual life you desire shines upon you. Seen by enemies and friends alike, you who were lost are found, and changed, and now bathed in Heavenly Light."

Contacts for *LAMAS Qi Gong* information and details

Website: www.cc-qi.com

Master: R. WILLIAMS
Swindon, England, UK (0776-691-9871)

Master: G. TONG
Delrey Beach, Florida, USA (561-715-9993)

Master: P. LAI
Ottawa, Canada (613-862-7505), (613-228-9211), (613-521-8222)

Master: J. GALAMAGA
Boynton Beach, Florida, USA (954-415-9569), (561-734-2342)

Professor: M. LIBOW
Boca Raton, Florida, USA (561-994-6446), (561-702-7212),
(561-350-8772), (561-994-4470)

Master: RISHA PENA
Berwyn, Illinois, USA (708-710-3416)

Master: E. EDWARDS
Mansfield, Nottinghamshire, England, UK (01623-646914)

Sifu: E. FOWLER
York, Pennsylvania, USA (717-968-1938)

Master: S. WONG
Illinois, USA (847-275-5990)

Professor: WAN YANG
Amsterdam, Holland, NL (3120-676-4128)

Sifu: A. LOBO
Dulwich. London, England, UK (0771-756771), (0208-6932140)

Master: STEVE CULLEN
Foxboro, Massachusetts, USA (508-543-5730)

Master: DONNELL JAKOBS
Seattle, Washington, USA (425-971-9222)

Master JACQUIE SHAM
Doncaster, England, UK (01302-538859)

Master ANDREW BEECH
Rotherham, Yorkshire, UK (07734-384388), (01709-519756)

Two Poems by A. S. Lowe

Is It?

Is it you or is it me?

Is it all that you see in me, not part of what lies within thee?

Am I not the reflection of what is within you, that which you hide?

Is it the shadow that moves in sympathy within which you reside?

Is it you or is it me that is a shadow or reflection?

Breathe deeply, think only of your breath's direction,

Where shallow breaths are toxic to the brain,

Breathing deeply regenerates one again.

Let your true and good self be an empty shell,

Display your light, unbidden, sound your life's bell.

Poems are written with great emotional empathy,

Thus let your breath prove the sweetest remedy.

Await not your ill met and untimely death,

Life is to be continued, take another inward breath.

My breath deeply taken and with great energy is sent,

Make safe of you is my sole intent.

Stress Gone

Open your mind like a fragrant flower,
Your Stress gone within an hour.

Stress perceived, is vibrations that surrounds,
Presented and unasked for, but still abounds.

The message stop may be received quite sharp,
A mishap or setback an error on one's part.

An opportunity to listen to that inner voice,
Breathe deeply and relax is in itself a choice.

Mind to listen, perhaps to hear stress of.
Unwanted problems, beyond and above.

Spirit, if but to feel for seconds in a day,
Awareness and practice makes stress go away.

If for a moment, you pause and then wait,
A healthy body such time does create.

Listen, you will hear the beat of your heart,
Saying stop and breathe, we never should part.

Listen to your breath it would have shown,
Out of the window, stress would have flown.

*To Order LAMAS Qi Gong
Videos and Books*

The Lion's Tail postures are demonstrated
by Grandmaster Lowe in the DVD:

Eliminate Stress.
*Develop Peace and Inner Calm
Ancient Healing Art*

It is available for $47.95 Plus shipping and handling.

Running time approximately 60 minutes

For US orders, please contact:
info@atouchofchi.com • Master Gary Tong
johngalamaga@aol.com • Master John Galamaga

For international orders, please visit:
www.cc-qi.com

Other Titles of Interest From
Ibis Books and Nicolas Hays, Inc.

Sacred Journey, A Pilgrimage to the Stations of the Cross in Jerusalem. By Steven Brooke. Take an extraordinary inspirational journey in the very footsteps of Christ along the pathway known as the Stations of the Cross. ISBN 978-0-89254-163-8 • 80 pages • 6 x 9 • Deluxe Hardcover • $21.95

Dervish Yoga for Health and Longevity, The Seven Major Arkanas. By Idris Lahore, Ennea Griffith, and Emma Thyloch. Details the seven fundamental arkana, or sacred exercises, of Samadeva, which are similar to the movements of yoga, T'ai Chi Ch'uan, and dance. ISBN: 0-89254-131-8 • 200 Pages • Illustrated • 7" x 10" • Paperback • $16.95

Way of the Small Why Less is Truly More. By Michael Gellert. Explores the principals of a sound, wholesome existence for both the individual and society. ISBN: 978-0-89254-129-4 • 192 Pages • 5" x 7" • Paperback • $14.95

A Call to Compassion, Bringing Buddhist Practices of the Heart into the Soul of Psychology. By Aura Glaser. Foreword by Robert A.F. Thurman. Explores Buddhist teachings on compassion and the Mahayana commitment to the liberation of all sentient beings. ISBN: 0-89254-116-4 • 304 Pages • 6" x 9" • Paperback • $16.95

In Praise of the Goddess The Devimahatmya and Its Meaning. A new translation, with commentary, of the sacred Hindu scripture and its eight Angas This spiritual classic, the Devimahatmya, addresses the perennial questions of the nature of the universe, humankind, and divinity. ISBN: 0-89254-080-X • 416 Pages • 6" x 9" • Paperback • $22.95

The Veiling Brilliance. By Devadatta Kali. This books tells the tale of three men—a king, a merchant, and a seer—but at its core is a revelation about the central tenets of goddess worship within an ancient religion. ISBN: 0-89254-128-8 • 256 Pages • 6" x 9" • Paperback • $18.95

Finding the Way. By Susan Montag. Foreword by Lon Milo DuQuette. Photography by Phillip Augusta. Written during the 6th century B.C.E., the *Tao Te Ching* is difficult for many Westerners to fathom as it attempts to describe what cannot be described: the way of the universe, its workings in human life, and how we can bring ourselves into harmony with it. ISBN: 0-89254-113-X • 128 Pages • 5 1/2" x 8 1/2" • Paperback. • $12.95

Edge of Certainty, Dilemmas on the Buddhist Path. By Peter Fenner Preface by Professor David Loy. This intriguing book challenges common conceptions and misconceptions about traveling the Buddhist path to enlightenment. ISBN: 0-89254-035-4 • 160 Pages • 5-1/2" x 8-1/2" • Paperback • $16.95

Essential Wisdom Teachings The Way to Inner Peace. By Peter & Penny Fenner. Provides a distillation of the profound wisdom teachings from many spiritual traditions. ISBN: 0-89254-053-2 • 176 Pages • 5-3/8" x 8-3/8" • Paperback • $16.95

Rassa Shastra. Inayat Khan on the Mysteries of Love, Sex, and Marriage. By Hazrat Inayat Khan. The author's classic books were among the first to bring Sufism to the West. They remain among the most important introductions Westerners have to the concepts of the ancient religious tradition. ISBN: 0-89254-071-0 • 96 Pages • 5" x 7" • Paperback • $18.95